ENGINEERING OF POLYSACCHARIDE MATERIALS

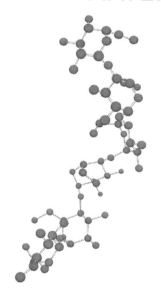

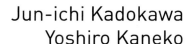

Jun-ichi Kadokawa
Yoshiro Kaneko

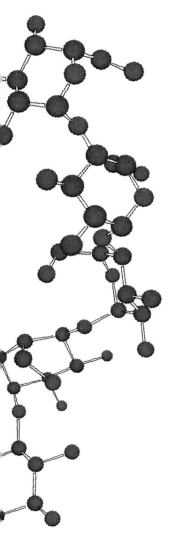

ENGINEERING OF POLYSACCHARIDE MATERIALS

By Phosphorylase-Catalyzed
Enzymatic Chain-Elongation

PAN STANFORD PUBLISHING

Published by

Pan Stanford Publishing Pte. Ltd.
Penthouse Level, Suntec Tower 3
8 Temasek Boulevard
Singapore 038988

Email: editorial@panstanford.com
Web: www.panstanford.com

British Library Cataloguing-in-Publication Data
A catalogue record for this book is available from the British Library.

ISBN 978-981-4364-45-4 (Hardcover)
ISBN 978-981-4364-46-1 (eBook)

Printed in the USA

Contents

Preface

Polysaccharides and related compounds are attracting much attention because of their potential for the applications as new functional materials in many research fields such as medicine, pharmaceutics, food, and cosmetics. Therefore, precision synthesis of new polysaccharides with well-defined structure is becoming increasingly important. For this purpose, enzymatic method is a very powerful tool because the reaction proceeds in a highly stereo- and regiocontrolled manner. Furthermore, the structurally complicated polysaccharides are synthesized by the enzymatic method. Among the enzymes that have been employed for the synthesis of polysaccharides, phosphorylase exhibits a potential to be used for the practical synthesis of α-glucans. However, this enzyme had not been used in the wide variety of polysaccharide researches compared with hydrolases (glycosidases and glycanases). Nowadays, however, the phosphorylase-catalyzed reaction (polymerization and chain elongation) has been well-known and a major category in the enzymatic synthesis of polysaccharides.

This book focuses on the advances in the practical synthesis of polysaccharides by the phosphorylase-catalyzed chain elongation on the basis of the viewpoint of polysaccharide engineering. Chapter 1 presents an overview of the importance of polysaccharides in materials engineering. The following three chapters deal with the fundamental aspects and characteristic features in the phosphorylase catalysis. The latter six chapters describe the practical synthesis of various polysaccharides materials by the phosphorylase catalysis, including polysaccharide-synthetic polymer hybrids, heteropolysaccharides, polysaccharide supramolecules, soft materials, and nanomaterials.

We believe that this book will provide an active source of information for research in polysaccharide science and engineering. Furthermore, this publication is directed to researchers and engineers in various academic and practical fields interested in the importance of polysaccharide materials.

We are indebted to the coworkers, whose names can be found in the references from our papers, for their enthusiastic collaborations. Finally, we wish to thank Mr. Stanford Chong, director and publisher, Pan Stanford Publishing, and his colleagues for their valuable contributions to this publication, which have been necessary in order to fruitfully accomplish the work.

Jun-ichi Kadokawa
Yoshiro Kaneko
February 2013

Chapter 1

Introduction

1.1 Important Features in Polysaccharides

Polysaccharides are one of the three major classes of biomacromolecules in the plant, animal, and microbial kingdom, which are vital materials for important *in vivo* functions, for example, providing an energy source, acting as a structural material, and conferring specific biological property [1,2]. They are structurally consisting of monosaccharide residues linked through glycosidic linkages. A glycosidic linkage is a type of covalent bond that joins a monosaccharide residue to another group, which may or may not be another saccharide residue. Polysaccharides have very complicated structures owing to not only a structurally variety of the monosaccharide residues but also the differences in stereo- and regio-types of the glycosidic linkages (Fig. 1.1) [2]. In contrast, the other two major biomacromolecules, i.e., nucleic acids and proteins, have relatively simple structures because these substrates are constructed by a type of specific linkage between several kinds of nucleotides and 20 kinds of amino acids, respectively (Fig. 1.1) [3]. A great variety of the polysaccharide structures contributes to serve a whole range of their functions in the host organism, and a subtle change in the structure of the monosaccharide unit or a type of glycosidic linkage has a profound effect on the properties and functions of the polysaccharides [4–6]. Therefore, synthesis of new

Engineering of Polysaccharide Materials: By Phosphorylase-Catalyzed Enzymatic Chain-Elongation
Jun-ichi Kadokawa and Yoshiro Kaneko
Copyright © 2013 Pan Stanford Publishing Pte. Ltd.
ISBN 978-981-4364-45-4 (Hardcover), ISBN 978-981-4364-46-1 (eBook)
www.panstanford.com

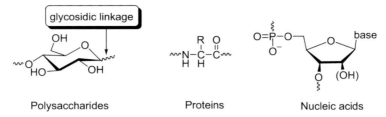

Polysaccharides   Proteins   Nucleic acids

Figure 1.1   Typical unit structures of polysaccharides, proteins, and nucleic acids.

polysaccharide compounds has attracted much attention because of their potential to apply as practical materials in the field of medicine, pharmaceutics, cosmetics, and food industries.

Cellulose, starch, and chitin are the most representative polysaccharides in nature (Fig. 1.2). Cellulose is the most abundant organic substance on the earth, which is composed of β-(1→4)-linked glucose residues [7]. It has been a symbolic molecule in polymers and macromolecules, and so far, various fundamental and practical studies on cellulose have been carried out, which concern its structure, chemical and physical properties, biosynthesis, and morphology. Starch is composed of both amylose with a linear structure and amylopectin with a branched structure [8]. The former consists of glucose residues linked through α-(1→4)-glycosidic linkages and the latter is composed of a linear chain of α-(1→4)-glycosidic linkages, interlinked by α-(1→6)-glycosidic linkages. Chitin is the second most abundant biological macromolecule on the earth after cellulose, which is found as a skeletal component of invertebrates. Chitin is composed of *N*-acetyl-D-glucosamine (GlcNAc) residues linked through β-(1→4)-glycosidic linkages [9,10].

Chemical synthesis of the polysaccharide was first performed by an attempt of cellulose synthesis in 1941 [11]. Then, attempts have been made to produce cellulose-type polysaccharides by traditional polymerization of glucose derivatives. For example, polycondensation of a glucose monomer, where hydroxy groups of 2-, 3-, and 6- positions were protected, was performed in the presence of P_2O_{10} to give the glucose polymer [12]. Although the authors claimed that the product had cellulose structure, definite evidence of the stereochemistry of glycosidic linkages, i.e., β-(1→4)-fashion, in the product was not sufficiently obtained. Since then, many efforts on polymerization had been devoted to chemical synthesis of polysaccharides with

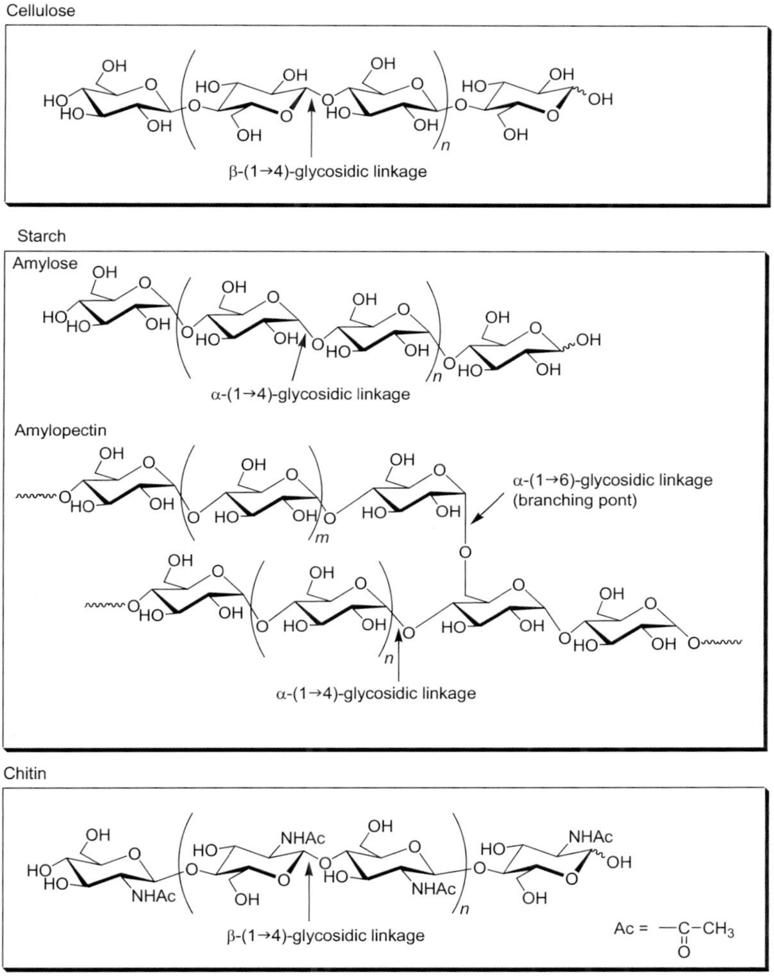

Cellulose

β-(1→4)-glycosidic linkage

Starch

Amylose

α-(1→4)-glycosidic linkage

Amylopectin

α-(1→6)-glycosidic linkage (branching pont)

α-(1→4)-glycosidic linkage

Chitin

β-(1→4)-glycosidic linkage

Ac = —C—CH₃ (O)

Figure 1.2   Structures of cellulose, starch, and chitin.

well-defined structure, but only a few approaches successfully led to the production of such polysaccharides. One approach is cationic ring-opening polymerization of anhydrosugar monomers [13]. After many attempts for this polymerization using various anhydrosugar monomers have been made, cellulose with degree of polymerization (DP) equal to 19.3 was synthesized by the cationic ring-opening polymerization of 3,6-di-*O*-benzyl-α-D-glucose 1,2,4-orthopivalate and the subsequent removal of the protective groups [14]. However, cationic ring-opening polyaddition of sugar oxazoline monomers derived from GlcNAc derivatives gave aminopolysaccharides with relatively controlled structures [15]. For example, a 3,6-*O*-dibenzylated sugar oxazoline monomer was polymerized with acid catalyst via ring-opening addition to give a dibenzyl chitin with DP is ca. 13 [16]. Then, removal of benzyl groups was carried out to give chitin [17]. However, complete deprotection did not take place. Because sugar monomers with protective groups have to be employed for the chemical synthesis of polysaccharides by polymerization, subsequent deprotection process is necessarily conducted to give free polysaccharides. Furthermore, perfect stereocontrol of glycosidic linkages has not often been achieved.

On the basis of the aforementioned backgrounds and viewpoints, almost in the past two decades, an enzymatic approach as a superior method to the traditional chemical one has been employed for the synthesis of polysaccharides with highly stereo- and regioselectivities [18–23].

1.2 Concept in Synthesis of Polysaccharides

Polysaccharides are produced by the repeated glycosylations of a glycosyl donor with a glycosyl acceptor to form a glycosidic linkage [24–26]. Figure 1.3 shows a typical schematic reaction of glycosylation for possible formation of a disaccharide. For the design of the substrates, an anomeric carbon (C1) of the glycosyl donor is activated by introducing a leaving group (X), and a hydroxy group in the glycosyl acceptor, which participates in the reaction, is employed as a free form, whereas other hydroxy groups in both the glycosyl donor and acceptor are protected. There are two important selectivities that should be controlled to form the glycosidic linkages. Because two possible geometric isomers, namely, α- and β-isomers, are conceived, the control of formation in such two glycosidic linkages, i.e., stereoselectivity, is one of the two important selectivities in the glycosylation. The other selectivity is regioselectivity. Monosaccharide has multiple hydroxy groups that participate in the formation of the glycosidic linkage. For example, glucose has four alcoholic hydroxy groups, excluding a hemiacetalic hydroxy group at C1 position, which can participate in the glycosylation. In the glycosylation using the glycosyl donor and acceptor derived from glucose, α- and β-isomers arise with respect to stereoselectivity of the anomeric carbon, and four isomers are conceivable with respect to regioselectivity owing to the four hydroxy groups in the acceptor. Thus, the glycosylation using the two glucose substrates involves a possibility for the production of eight isomers for the glucose dimer (Fig. 1.4). The large numbers of isomers for the oligosaccharides composed of glucose residues are theoretically calculated [25]. Among the multiple fashions of the glycosidic linkages, only one kind of the linkage must be constructed to produce polysaccharides with well-defined structure on the basis of the aforementioned two important selectivities in the glycosylation.

For stereo- and regioselective construction of the glycosidic linkage, a leaving group, protective groups, a catalyst, and a solvent should appropriately be selected. Over the past century, the reaction control in the glycosylation has been one of the main research areas in the carbohydrate chemistry. Although many chemical glycosylations using various glycosyl donors, acidic catalysts,

Figure 1.3   Reaction manner of glycosylation.

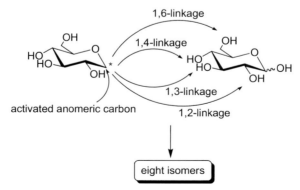

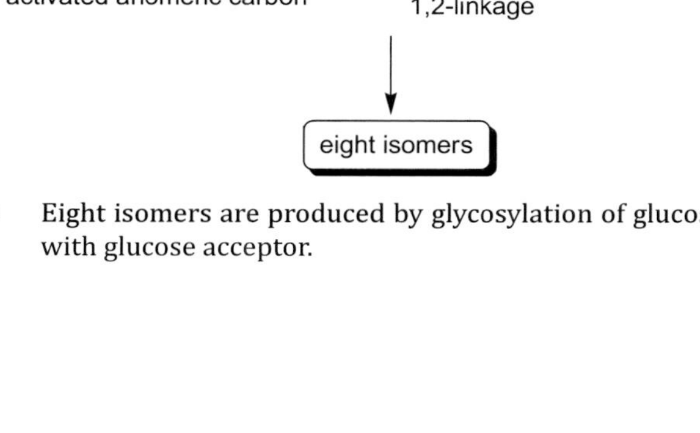

Figure 1.4   Eight isomers are produced by glycosylation of glucose donor with glucose acceptor.

protective groups, and solvent systems have been developed for the stereoselective construction of the glycosidic linkages, the perfection in the selectivity still remains as a challenging problem [27]. As appeared in two representative natural polysaccharides, i.e., cellulose and starch, the importance in fashions of the glycosidic linkages in the polysaccharides is significant for their functions [2]. Cellulose and starch are composed of the same structural unit, i.e., the glucose unit, but linked through the different β-(1→4)- and α-(1→4)-glycosidic linkages, respectively. Owing to the difference in such stereochemistry of glycosidic linkages in cellulose and starch, their roles in nature are completely different; the former is a structural material and the latter acts as the energy source. In the synthesis of polysaccharides, therefore, perfect control of stereo- and regiochemistries in the glycosidic linkages is strictly demanded. Furthermore, the chemical glycosylations require the protection–deprotection processes of the hydroxy groups. During the multiple reaction steps for the synthesis of polysaccharides via the chemical glycosylations, therefore, undesired side-reactions often take place.

To develop a superior method for the synthesis of polysaccharides, the *in vitro* approach by enzymatic catalysis has been significantly investigated [18–23]. Enzymes have several remarkable catalytic properties compared with other types of catalyst in terms of the stereo- and regioselectivities. In addition, enzymatic reaction is one of the most promising basic technologies with a simple operation under mild conditions, eliminating undesirable side-reactions. Thus, the next chapter describes the general scope for an enzymatic method in polysaccharide synthesis.

References

1. Berg, J. M., Tymoczko, L. J., and Stryer, L. (2006). *Biochemistry*, 6th International Ed., Chapter 11 "Carbohydrates" (W. H. Freeman & Co., NY).

2. Schuerch, C. (1986). *Encyclopedia of Polymer Science and Engineering*, 2nd Ed., eds. Mark, H. F., Bilkales, N., and Overberger, C. G., Vol. 13, "Polysaccharides" (John Wiley & Sons, NY), pp. 87–162.

3. McMurry, J., Castellion, M. E., Ballantine, D. S., and Hoeger, C. A. (2009). *Fundamentals of General, Organic, and Biological Chemistry*, 6th Ed. (Prentice Hall Inc., NJ).

4. Ernst, B., Hart, G. W., and Sinäy, P. (eds) (2000). *Carbohydrates in Chemistry and Biology* (Wiley-VCH, Weinheim).

5. Fraser-Reid, B. O., Tatsuta, K., Thiem, J., Coté, G. L., Flitsch, S., Ito, Y., Kondo, H., Nishimura, S.-I., and Yu, B. eds. (2008). *Glycoscience*, 2nd Ed. (Springer, Berlin).

6. Varki, A., Cummings, R. D., Esko, J. D., Freeze, H. H., Stanley, P., Bertozzi, C. R., Hart, G. W., and Etzler, M. E. eds. (2009). *Essentials of Glycobiology*, 2nd Ed. (Cold Spring Harbor Laboratory Press, NY).

7. Klemm, D., Heublein, B., Fink, H. P., and Bohn, A. (2005). Cellulose: Fascinating biopolymers and sustainable raw material, *Angew. Chem., Int. Ed.*, **44**, pp. 3358–3393.

8. Lenz, R. W. (1993). Biodegradable polymers, *Adv. Polym. Sci.*, **107**, pp. 1–40.

9. Muzzarelli, R. A. A. (1977). *Chitin* (Pergamon Press, Oxford).

10. Muzzarelli, R. A. A., Jeuniaux, C., and Gooday, G. W. eds. (1986). *Chitin in Nature and Technology* (Plenum Press, NY).

11. Schlubach, H. H., and Lührs, E. (1941). Einwirkung von chlorwasserstoff auf glucose. synthese eines polyglucosans, *Liebigs Ann. Chem.*, **547**, pp. 73–85.

12. Husemann, Von E., and Müller, G. J. M. (1966). Über die synthese unverzweigter polysaccharide, *Makromol. Chem.*, **91**, pp. 212–230.

13. Schuerch, C. (1973). Systematic approaches to the chemical synthesis of polysaccharides, *Acc. Chem. Res.*, **6**, pp. 184–191.

14. Nakatsubo, F., Kamitakahara, H., and Hori, M. (1996). Cationic ring-opening polymerization of 3,6-di-*O*-benzyl-α-D-glucose 1,2,4-orthopivalate and the first chemical synthesis of cellulose, *J. Am. Chem. Soc.*, **118**, pp. 1677–1681.

15. Kadokawa, J., Tagaya, H., and Chiba, K. (2001). Synthesis of linear and hyperbranched stereoregular aminopolysaccharides by oxazoline glycosylation, In *Polymeric Drugs & Drug Delivery Systems* (Ottenbrite, R. M., and Kim, S. W., eds), Technomic Publishing Company, Inc., Lancaster, Chapter 18, pp. 251–264.

16. Kadokawa, J., Watanabe, Y., Karasu, M., Tagaya, H., and Chiba, K. (1996). Synthesis of a dibenzylchitin-type polysaccharide by acid-catalyzed polymerization, *Macromol. Rapid Commun.*, **17**, pp. 367–372.

17. Kadokawa, J., Kasai, S., Watanabe, Y., Karasu, M., Tagaya, H., and Chiba, K. (1997). Synthesis of natural- and non-natural-type aminopolysaccharides: 2-Acetamido-2-deoxy-β-D-glucopyranan

derivatives by acid-catalyzed polymerization of 2-methyl(3,6- and 3,4-di-*O*-benzyl-1,2-dideoxy-α-ᴅ-glucopyrano)-[2,1-*d*]-2-oxazolines involving stereoregular glycosylation, *Macromolecules*, **30**, pp. 8212–8217.

18. Kobayashi, S., Uyama, H., and Kimura, S. (2001). Enzymatic polymerization, *Chem. Rev.*, **101**, pp. 3793–3818.

19. Kobayashi, S. (2005). Challenge of synthetic cellulose, *J. Polym. Sci., Part A: Polym. Chem.*, **43**, pp. 693–710.

20. Kobayashi, S. (2007). New development of polysaccharide synthesis via enzymatic polymerization, *Proc. Jpn. Acad., Ser. B*, **83**, pp. 215–247.

21. Kobayashi, S., and Makino, A. (2009). Enzymatic polymer synthesis: An opportunity for green polymer chemistry, *Chem. Rev.*, **109**, pp. 5288–5353.

22. Kadokawa, J., and Kobayashi, S. (2010). Polymer synthesis by enzymatic catalysis, *Curr. Opin. Chem. Biol.*, **14**, pp. 145–153.

23. Kadokawa, J. (2011). Precision polysaccharide synthesis catalyzed by enzymes, *Chem. Rev.*, **111**, pp. 4308–4345.

24. Paulsen, H. (1982). Advances in selective chemical syntheses of complex oligosaccharides, *Angew. Chem., Int. Ed. Engl.*, **21**, pp. 155–173.

25. Schmidt, R. R. (1986). New methods of the synthesis of glycosides and oligosaccharides: Are there alternative to the Koenigs–Knorr methods?, *Angew. Chem., Int. Ed. Engl.*, **25**, pp. 212–235.

26. Toshima, K., and Tatsuta, K. (1993). Recent progress in *O*-glycosylation methods and its application to natural products synthesis, *Chem. Rev.*, **93**, pp. 1503–1531.

27. Mydock, L. K., and Demchenko, A. V. (2010). Mechanism of chemical *O*-glycosylation: From early studies to recent discoveries, *Org. Biomol. Chem.*, **8**, pp. 497–510.

Chapter 2

General Scope for Enzymatic Tools in Engineering of Polysaccharide Materials

2.1 Characteristic Features of Enzymatic Reactions for Synthesis of Polysaccharides

All the biosubstances, including polysaccharides, are produced *in vivo* by enzymatic catalysis. Because enzymatic catalysis has attracted much attention and grown in importance in biochemistry, organic chemistry, and polymer chemistry, fundamental research studies on enzymes and enzymatic reactions are still one of the main topics in these research fields. Enzymes are generally categorized into six main classes, which are oxidoreductases (EC 1), transferases (EC 2), hydrolases (EC 3), lyases (EC 4), isomerases (EC 5), and ligases (EC 6) [1]. In the main classes, two enzymes, i.e., transferases and hydrolases, have been practically applied as catalysts for the *in vitro* enzymatic synthesis of polysaccharides [2,3]. In general, enzymatic catalysis has the following advantageous characteristics: (1) progress of reactions under mild conditions, (2) high selectivities of stereo-, regio-, enantio-, and chemoregulations leading to structurally controlled products, and (3) large turnover numbers. These characteristics of enzymatic catalyses induce the following expectations for the precision synthesis of polysaccharides: (1) perfect control of stereo- and regioselectivities in glycosidic linkages, (2) production of new

Engineering of Polysaccharide Materials: By Phosphorylase-Catalyzed Enzymatic Chain-Elongation
Jun-ichi Kadokawa and Yoshiro Kaneko
Copyright © 2013 Pan Stanford Publishing Pte. Ltd.
ISBN 978-981-4364-45-4 (Hardcover), ISBN 978-981-4364-46-1 (eBook)
www.panstanford.com

nonnatural polysaccharides, and (3) achievement of green processes without the use of harmful catalysts such as strong acids or bases and heavy metals and the formation of byproducts.

Furthermore, the following two aspects should be emphasized further as fundamental and important characteristics in enzymatic reactions. The first is a "key and lock" theory proposed by Fischer in 1984 [4], which points out the relation of enzyme to native substrate. The theory implies that a specific substrate and an enzyme correspond strictly in a 1:1 fashion like a key and lock relationship in biosynthetic pathways. In the enzyme–substrate complex, the substrate is located in the enzyme with geometrical adaptation, leading to a product with perfect structural control. However, the key and lock relationship observed for *in vitro* enzymatic reactions is not absolutely strict in many cases. Enzymes often have loose specificity for recognition of the substrate structure and can insert with not only a natural substrate but also a nonnatural one having the similar structure as that of the former. In the case of *in vitro* enzymatic synthesis of polysaccharides via nonbiosynthetic pathways, the nonnatural substrate can be employed for the enzymatic catalysis. The substrate is recognized by an enzyme to form a complex, resulting in the progress of the desired reaction (Fig. 2.1).

The second characteristic for the enzymatic reaction is an energy diagram. Pauling demonstrated in 1946 the reason why enzymatic reactions proceed under the mild conditions [5]. The formation of the enzyme–substrate complex stabilizes the transition state and

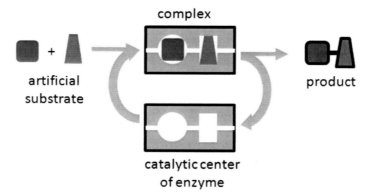

Figure 2.1   The key and lock relationship for *in vitro* nonbiosynthetic pathway.

lowers the activation energy compared with the nonenzymatic case.

Similar to the general glycosylation, enzymatic formation of a glycosidic linkage between C-1 atom of a monosaccharide and one of the hydroxy groups of the other monosaccharide can be realized by the reaction of an activated glycosyl donor and a glycosyl acceptor (Fig. 2.2) [6]. First, the glycosyl donor is recognized by an enzyme to form a glycosyl–enzyme intermediate (or transition state). Then, the intermediate is attacked by the hydroxy group of the glycosyl acceptor, giving a glycoside. On the basis of the above characteristics of the enzymatic reactions, it has generally been well accepted that enzymatic glycosylation is a very powerful tool for the stereo- and regioselective construction of the glycosidic linkages under the mild conditions, where a glycosyl donor and a glycosyl acceptor can be employed in their unprotected forms, leading to the direct formation of unprotected saccharide chains in aqueous media [7]. Thus, repetition of the enzymatic glycosylations forms polysaccharides with well-defined structure. As mentioned earlier, enzymes involved in the synthesis of polysaccharides are categorized into two main classes: hydrolytic enzymes (hydrolases) and glycosyltransferases (Fig. 2.3). The latter is precisely subclassified further into synthetic enzymes (Leloir glycosyltransferases) [3], phosphorolytic enzymes (phosphorylases) [8], and others [9].

Phosphorylases, which this book focuses on as a catalyst for the efficient production of polysaccharide materials, catalyze phosphorolytic cleavage of a glycosidic linkage in the saccharide chain in the presence of inorganic phosphate to produce glycose 1-phosphate and the saccharide chain with one smaller DP. Because the bond energy of the produced phosphate is comparable with that of the glycosidic linkage, the phosphorylase-catalyzed reactions exhibit reversible nature. Therefore, phosphorylases can

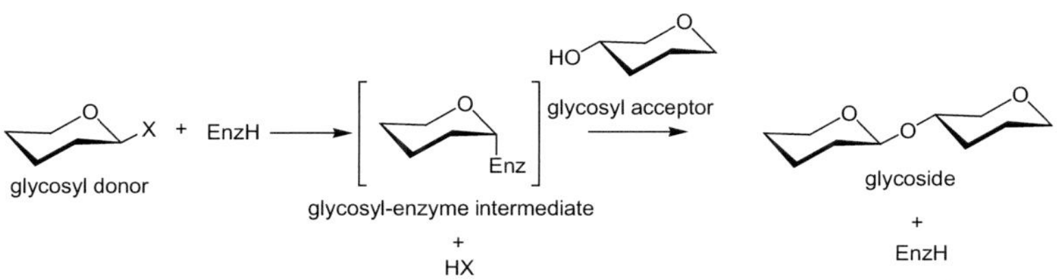

Figure 2.2 General reaction scheme for enzymatic glycosylation.

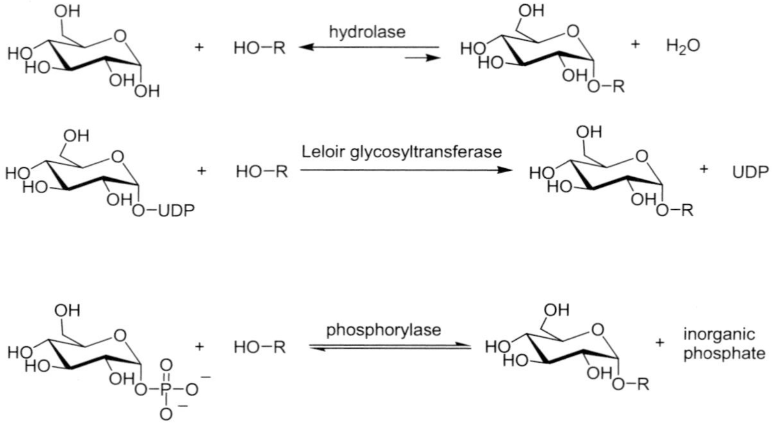

Figure 2.3   Typical enzymes involved in the synthesis of polysaccharides.

be employed in the practical synthesis of saccharide chains via glycosylation. In such glycosylations catalyzed by phophorylases, the glycose 1-phosphates are used as a glycosyl donor and the glycose unit is transferred from the substrate to a nonreducing end of an appropriate glycosyl acceptor to form a stereo- and regiocontrolled glycosidic linkage accompanied with the production of inorganic phosphate.

Leloir glycosyltransferases are biologically important because they perform the role of synthesizing saccharide chains *in vivo* [10]. The reactions of the enzymes are irreversible in the synthetic direction because of the requirement for cleavage of the high-energy linkage of the glycosyl nucleotide substrates. However, Leloir glycosyltransferases are generally transmembrane-type proteins, present in nature in very small amounts, and unstable for isolation and purification. Therefore, the enzymes are expensive and hardly available. Hydrolases have been frequently employed in the hydrolysis of polysaccharides, which are industrially important in the utilization of natural polysaccharides such as starch. The hydrolase catalysis using natural polysaccharides readily proceed in the way to hydrolysis under the normal conditions in aqueous media. However, when an enzyme–substrate complex is formed, hydrolases catalyzing hydrolysis *in vivo* are able to catalyze a glycosylation *in vitro* to produce the saccharide chains. This view is based on a hypothesis that the structures of transition states are very close in both *in vivo* and *in vitro* reactions [11–14]. The other enzyme in glycosyltransferases, which are often employed in the synthesis of polysaccharides, is sucrase-type enzyme [9]. This class of enzymes is the glycosyltransferase that is highly specialized in transfer either of a glucose or of a fructose moiety in a substrate of sucrose. Thus, the sucrase-type enzymes form either glucose-based polysaccharides (glucans) or fructose-based polysaccharides (fructans) of different types with respect to glycosidic linkages and side chains. Before going into the main topic of this book, which is the phosphorylase-catalyzed enzymatic chain elongation, herein in this chapter, the synthesis of polysaccharides catalyzed by hydrolases and sucrase-type enzymes are briefly overviewed.

2.2 Synthesis of Polysaccharides Catalyzed by Hydrolases

For the synthesis of polysaccharides by the polymerization catalyzed by hydrolases, the substrates (monomers) should be designed as the structure of a transition state analogue [11–14]. On the basis of this concept, two types of monomers, i.e., glycosyl fluorides and sugar oxazolines, have been designed to be efficiently recognized by hydrolases [15,16]. The anomeric carbon is activated by introducing fluoride or an oxazoline group (1,2-oxazoline derived from 2-acetamido-2-deoxysugar), giving the substrates that have structures close to a transition state of enzymatic reactions and efficiently form the enzyme–substrate complexes. In the two types of hydrolases, i.e., endo- and exotypes, the former has been found to be an efficient catalyst for the enzymatic synthesis of polysaccharides. Endotype hydrolases (endoglycosidases) cleave a glycosidic linkage of the inner unit of polysaccharides. The shapes at the catalytic domain of endoglycosidases look like cleft. Glycosyl fluorides have been found to act as a glycosyl donor for enzymatic glycosylation catalyzed by endoglycosidases. The merit using glycosyl fluorides as the glycosyl donor originates from the unique properties of a fluorine atom [17]. A first point is that the size of a fluorine atom is comparable to that of a hydroxy group and it can accordingly be accepted by an active site of an enzyme. Second, in glycosyl halides, only glycosyl fluoride is stable as an unprotected form, which is necessary for the enzymatic reactions in aqueous media. A third point is that a C–F linkage in the glycosyl fluoride can be cleaved readily because of a good leaving group of the fluoride. However, sugar oxazolines with unprotected form were also found to be an efficient glycosyl donor for enzymatic glycosylation [7].

By enzymatic polymerization, using glycosyl fluorides, cellulose, amylose, xylan, and related polysaccharides have been synthesized [11–16], and enzymatic polymerization using sugar oxazolines produced chitin, hyaluronan, chondroitin, and related aminopolysaccharides [11–16,18–20]. The former proceeds via the polycondensation through leaving hydrogen fluoride, whereas the ring-opening polyaddition is conceived in the polymerization manner of the latter case.

The synthesis of cellulose was achieved in 1991 by enzymatic polymerization of β-cellobiosyl fluoride catalyzed by cellulase (Fig. 2.4a) [21]. The polymerization proceeded via polycondensation with liberating hydrogen fluoride, where the monomer behaved as both the glycosyl donor and acceptor for cellulase. Mixing organic solvents with buffer was necessary as a medium to prevent the hydrolysis of produced cellulose by cellulase catalysis. Because the suppression of the hydrolysis was incomplete as long as the wild-type cellulase was used, the mutant cellulase was designed such that the polymerization would take place more efficiently [22]. A novel approach for the enzymatic polycondensation using cellobiose as a starting substrate without activation of the anomeric carbon was reported [23]. This was achieved using a cellulase/surfactant complex as the catalyst in a nonaqueous LiCl/N,N-dimethylacetamide system. Cellobiose was polymerized by the catalyst of the complex to give cellulose with high molecular weight. The enzymatic polymerization of α-maltosyl fluoride catalyzed by an endotype enzyme, α-amylase, which catalyzes random hydrolysis of α-(1→4)-glucan chain, proceeded in a mixed solvent of methanol/buffer to give amylose oligomers (Fig. 2.4b) [24]. β-Xylobiosyl fluoride was designed as a monomer for the synthesis of xylan, a β-(1→4)-linked xylose polysaccharide, by the enzymatic polymerization catalyzed by cellulase, because its commercial-grade enzyme has been known to show xylanase activity (Fig. 2.4c) [25]. Consequently, the cellulase-catalyzed enzymatic polymerization of this monomer proceeded in a mixed solvent of acetonitorile/buffer to give a synthetic xylan.

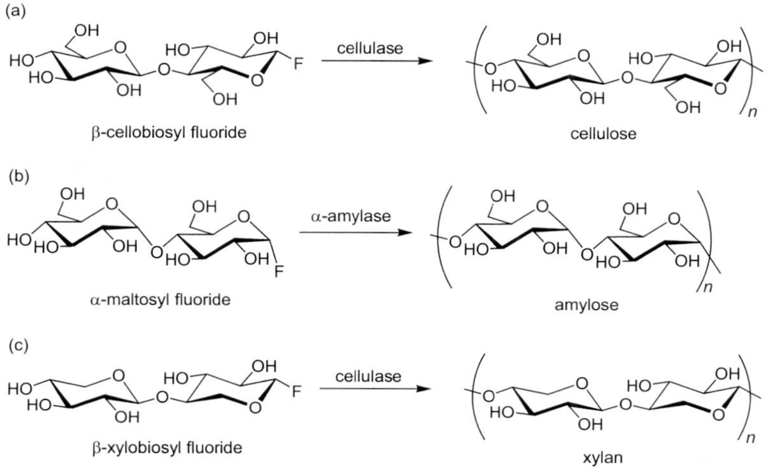

(a)

β-cellobiosyl fluoride   cellulose

(b)

α-maltosyl fluoride   amylose

(c)

β-xylobiosyl fluoride   xylan

Figure 2.4   Hydrolase-catalyzed polymerization of glycosyl fluorides to synthetic cellulose (a), amylose (b), and xylan (c).

In vitro synthesis of chitin was first reported by utilizing chitinase as a catalyst [26]. The chitinase-catalyzed enzymatic polymerization of a *N,N'*-diacetylchitobiose oxazoline monomer proceeded via ring-opening polyaddition under weak alkaline conditions, giving a synthetic chitin (Fig. 2.5a). The process of the higher ordered self-assembly of the synthetic chitin during the enzymatic polymerization was directly observed by phase-contrast and polarization microscopes with SEM and TEM [27]. Hyaluronidase has shown a wide spectrum of catalysis for the ring-opening polyaddition of a variety of sugar oxazoline monomers, controlling stereochemistry and regioselectivity perfectly to provide many natural and nonnatural glycosaminoglycans [19]. For example, hyaluronan, which is a linear polysaccharide having a repeating unit of β-(1→3)-GlcNAc-β-(1→4)-GlcA (GlcA, glucuronic acid) was produced by the hyaluronidase-catalyzed polymerization of a GlcA-β-(1→3)-GlcNAc oxazoline monomer (Fig. 2.5b) [28]. Chondroitin, other glycosaminoglycan, whose structure difference from hyaluronan is the difference in stereochemistry of C-4 in hexosamine unit. Therefore, GlcA-β-(1→3)-GalNAc oxazoline monomer (GalNAc, *N*-acetyl-D-galactosamine) was designed for the synthesis of chondroitin via the hyaluronidase-catalyzed ring-opening polyaddition (Fig. 2.5c) [29].

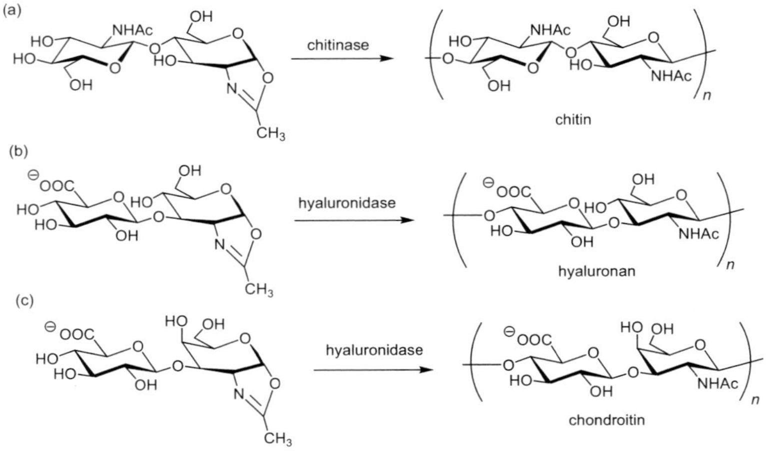

Figure 2.5 Hydrolase-catalyzed polymerization of sugar oxazolines to synthetic chitin (a), hyaluronan (b), and chondroitin (c).

2.3 Synthesis of Polysaccharides Catalyzed by Sucrase-Type Enzymes

Non-Leloir-type glycosyltransferases that use sucrose as a substrate are able to catalyze the synthesis of polysaccharides in high yields under kinetic control, even in dilute aqueous solution of sucrose [9]. Most enzymes of this class highly specialize in transfer of either the glucose or the fructose moiety of sucrose, giving glucose-based polysaccharides (glucans) or fructose-based polysaccharides (fructans) of different types with respect to glycosidic linkages and side chains. The simplified reaction schemes are shown as follows:
Glucosyltransferases

n sucrose → glucan + n fructose

Fluctosyltransferases

n sucrose → fructan + n glucose

The enzymes of this group are often called sucrase-type enzymes, i.e., glucosyltransferases are glucansucrases and fructosyltransferases are fructansucrases.

Glucansucrases are typically extracellular enzymes, which are produced mainly by lactic acid bacteria [30]. Dextran-, mutan-, alternan-, reuteran-, and amylosucrases produce dextran (α-(1→6)-glucan), mutan (α-(1→3)-glucan), alternan (α-(1→3)-*alt*-α-(1→6)-glucan), reutinan (α-(1→4)-*co*-α-(1→6)-glucan), and amylose (α-(1→4)-glucan), respectively (Fig. 2.6) [31]. Furthermore, the modifications with respect to the glycosidic linkage pattern in polysaccharide synthesis have been investigated. Amylosucrase is the most extensively studied glucansucrase. Recombinant amylosucrase was used to synthesize amylose from sucrose without use of an acceptor [32]. The recombinant amylosucrase was also used for the chain-elongation reaction in the presence of glycogen as an acceptor [33]. The morphology and structure of the resulting insoluble products were shown to strongly depend on the initial sucrose/glycogen ratio.

Fructansucrases transfer the fructose units of sucrose onto polysaccharides or appropriate acceptors with release of glucose. Fructans, thus produced, are either levan composed of β-(2→6)-fructan by levansucrase catalysis or inulin composed of β-(2→1)-fructan by inulinsucrase catalysis (Fig. 2.6) [31]. Sucrose analogues, which are nonnatural substrates with a similar glycosidic linkage to sucrose, have been used for the synthesis of new poly- and oligosaccharides by catalysis of sucrase-type enzymes. For this purpose, a whole range of sucrose analogues have been prepared. A wide range of fructansucrases recognize most of them, giving rise to novel poly- or oligosaccharides [34,35].

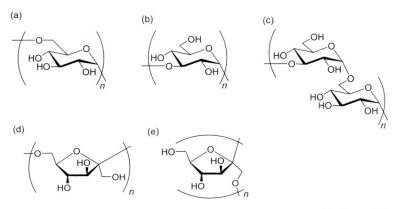

Figure 2.6 Structures of dextran (a), mutan (b), alternan (c), levan (d), and inulin (e).

References

1. Webb, E. C. (ed.) (1992). *Enzyme Nomenclature 1992, Recommendations of the NCIUBMB on the Nomenclature and Classification of Enzymes* (International Union of Biochemistry and Molecular Biology, Academic Press, San Diego).

2. Murata, T., and Usui, T. (2000). Enzymatic synthesis of important oligosaccharide units involved in N- and O-linked glycans, *Trends Glycosci. Glycotechnol.*, **12**, pp. 161–174.

3. Taniguchi, N., Honke, K., and Fukuda, M. (eds) (2002). *Handbook of Glycosyltransferases and Related Genes* (Springer, Tokyo).

4. Fischer, E. (1894). Einfluss der configuration auf die wirkung der enzyme, *Ber. Dtsch. Chem. Ges.*, **27**, pp. 2985–2993.

5. Kollman, P. A., Kuhn, B., Donini, O., Perakyla, M., Stanton, R., and Bakowies, D. (2001). Elucidating the nature of enzyme catalysis utilizing a new twist on an old methodology: Quantum mechanical–free energy calculations on chemical reactions in enzymes and in aqueous solution, *Acc. Chem. Res.*, **34**, pp. 72–79.

6. Shoda, S., Fujita, M., and Kobayashi, S. (1998). Glycanase-catalyzed synthesis of non-natural oligosaccharides, *Trends Glycosci. Glycotechnol.*, **10**, pp. 279–289.

7. Shoda, S., Izumi, R., and Fujita, M. (2003). Green process in glycotechnology, *Bull. Chem. Soc. Jpn.*, **76**, pp. 1–13.

8. Kitaoka, M., and Hayashi, K. (2002). Carbohydrate-processing phosphorolytic enzymes, *Trends Glycosci. Glycotechnol.*, **14**, pp. 35–50.

9. Seibel, J., Jördening, H.-J., and Buchholz, K. (2006). Glycosylation with activated sugars using glycosyltransferases and transglycosidases, *Biocatal. Biotranform.*, **24**, pp. 311–342.

10. Rupprath, C., Schumacher, T., and Elling, L. (2005). Nucleotide deoxysugars: Essential tools for the glycosylation engineering of novel bioactive compounds, *Curr. Med. Chem.*, **12**, pp. 1637–1675.

11. Kobayashi, S. (2007). New developments of polysaccharide synthesis via enzymatic polymerization, *Proc. Jpn. Acad. Ser. B*, **83**, pp. 215–247.

12. Kobayashi, S., and Makino, A. (2009). Enzymatic polymer synthesis: An opportunity for green polymer chemistry, *Chem. Rev.*, **109**, pp. 5288–5353.

13. Kadokawa, J., and Kobayashi, S. (2010). Polymer synthesis by enzymatic catalysis, *Curr. Opin. Chem. Biol.*, **14**, pp. 145–153.

14. Kadokawa, J. (2011). Precision polysaccharide synthesis catalyzed by enzymes, *Chem. Rev.*, **111**, pp. 4308–4345.

15. Kobayashi, S. (2005). Challenge of synthetic cellulose, *J. Polym. Sci., Part A: Polym. Chem.*, **43**, pp. 693–710.

16. Makino, A., and Kobayashi, S. (2010). Chemistry of 2-oxazolines: A crossing of cationic ring-opening polymerization and enzymatic ring-opening polyaddition, *J. Polym. Sci., Part A: Polym. Chem.*, **48**, pp. 1251–1270.

17. Kobayashi, S., Uyama, H., and Kimura, S. (2001). Enzymatic polymerization, *Chem. Rev.*, **101**, pp. 3793–3818.

18. Ohmae, M., Fujikawa, S., Ochiai, H., and Kobayashi, S. (2006). Enzyme-catalyzed synthesis of natural and unnatural polysaccharides, *J. Polym. Sci., Part A: Polym. Chem.*, **44**, pp. 5014–5027.

19. Kobayashi, S., Ohmae, M., Ochiai, H., and Fujikawa, S. (2006). A hyaruronidase supercatalyst for the enzymatic polymerization to synthesize glycosaminoglycans, *Chem. Eur. J.*, **12**, pp. 5962–5971.

20. Ohmae, M., Makino, A., and Kobayashi, S. (2007). Enzymatic polymerization to unnatural hybrid polysaccharides, *Macromol. Chem. Phys.*, **208**, pp. 1447–1457.

21. Kobayashi, S., Kashiwa, K., Kawasaki, T., and Shoda, S. (1991). Novel method for polysaccharide synthesis using an enzyme – The 1st *in vitro* synthesis of cellulose via a nonbiosynthetic path utilizing cellulase as catalyst, *J. Am. Chem. Soc.*, **113**, pp. 3079–3084.

22. Nakamura, I., Yoneda, H., Maeda, T., Makino, A., Ohmae, M., Sugiyama, J., Ueda, M., Kobayashi, S., and Kimura, S. (2005). Enzymatic polymerization behavior using cellulose-binding domain deficient endoglucanase II, *Macromol. Biosci.*, **5**, pp. 623–628.

23. Egusa, S., Kitaoka, T., Goto, M., and Wariishi, H. (2007). Synthesis of cellulose *in vitro* by using a cellulase/surfactant complex in a nonaqueous medium, *Angew. Chem., Int. Ed.*, **46**, pp. 2063–2065.

24. Kobayashi, S., Shimada, J., Kashiwa, K., and Shoda, S. (1992). Enzymatic polymerization of α-D-maltosyl fluoride utilizing α-amylase as the catalyst – A new approach for the synthesis of maltooligosaccharides, *Macromolecules*, **25**, pp. 3237–3241.

25. Kobayashi, S., Wen, X., and Shoda, S. (1996). Specific preparation of artificial xylan: A new approach to polysaccharide synthesis by using cellulase as catalyst, *Macromolecules*, **29**, pp. 2698–2700.

26. Kobayashi, S., Kiyosada, T., and Shoda, S. (1996). Synthesis of artificial chitin: Irreversible catalytic behavior of a glycosyl hydrolase through a

transition state analogue substrate, *J. Am. Chem. Soc.*, **118**, pp. 13113–13114.

27. Sakamoto, J., Sugiyama, J., Kimura, S., Imai, T., Itoh, T., Watanabe, T., and Kobayashi, S. (2000). Artificial chitin spherulites composed of single crystalline ribbons of alpha-chitin via enzymatic polymerization, *Macromolecules*, **33**, pp. 4155–4160.

28. Kobayashi, S., Morii, H., Itoh, R., Kimura, S., and Ohmae, M. (2001). Enzymatic polymerization to artificial hyaluronan: A novel method to synthesize a glycosaminoglycan using a transition state analogue monomer, *J. Am. Chem. Soc.*, **123**, pp. 11825–11826.

29. Kobayashi, S., Fujikawa, S., and Ohmae, M. (2003). Enzymatic synthesis of chondroitin and its derivatives catalyzed by hyaluronidase, *J. Am. Chem. Soc.*, **125**, pp. 14357–14369.

30. Monchois, V., Willemot, R.-M., and Monsan, P. (1999). Glucansucrases: Mechanism of action and structure-function relationships, *FEMS Microbiol. Rev.*, **23**, pp. 131–151.

31. van Hijum, S. A. F. T., Kralj, S., Ozimek, L. K., Dijkhuizen, L., and van Geel-Schutten, I. G. H. (2006). Structure-function relationships of glucansucrase and fructansucrase enzymes from lactic acid bacteria, *Microbiol. Mol. Biol. Rev.*, **70**, pp. 157–176.

32. Potocki-Véronèse, G., Putaux, J.-L., Dupeyre, D., Albenne, C., Remaud-Simeon, M., Monsan, P., and Buleon, A. (2005). Amylose synthesized *in vitro* by amylosucrase: Morphology, structure, and properties, *Biomacromolecules*, **6**, pp. 1000–1011.

33. Putaux, J.-L., Potocki-Véronèse, G., Remaud-Simeon, M., and Buleon, A. (2006). α-D-glucan-based dendritic nanoparticles prepared by *in vitro* enzymatic chain extension of glycogen, *Biomacromolecules*, **7**, pp. 1720–1728.

34. Beine, R., Moraru, R., Nimtz, M., Na'amnieh, S., Pawlowski, A., Buchholz, K., and Seibel, J. (2008). Synthesis of novel fructooligosaccharides by substrate and enzyme engineering, *J. Biotechnol.*, **138**, pp. 33–41.

35. Homann, A., and Seibel, J. (2009). Towards tailor-made oligosaccharides-chemo-enzymatic approaches by enzyme and substrate engineering, *Appl. Microbiol. Biotechnol.*, **83**, pp. 209–216.

Chapter 3

Phosphorylase-Catalyzed Enzymatic Glycosylation

3.1   Fundamental Features of Phosphorylases

Various phosphorylases have been known, as summarized in Table 3.1, and all of them catalyze an exo-wise phosphorolysis of the glycosidic linkage at the nonreducing end in the presence of an inorganic phosphate (Fig. 3.1) [1,2]. The enzymes are named using a combination of "the name of the substrate and phosphorylase." The phosphorylases are generally classified by the anomeric forms of the glycosidic linkages in the substrates that are phosphorolyzed or by the anomeric forms of the glycose 1-phosphates that are produced. The other way employed to classify phosphorylases is describing them in terms of the anomeric retention or inversion in the reaction. The stereo- and regiospecificities of phosphorylases are very strict, and they catalyze the phosphorolysis of the specific type of glycosidic linkages. The characteristics are important in the exploitation of phosphorylases for the synthesis of oligo- and polysaccharides with well-defined structure via the reverse reaction of the phosphorolysis. Several phosphorylases can be employed for the synthesis of polysaccharides or even oligosaccharides with relatively high DPs, but other phosphorylases recognize only disaccharide substrates and catalyze the reversible phosphorolysis

Engineering of Polysaccharide Materials: By Phosphorylase-Catalyzed Enzymatic Chain-Elongation
Jun-ichi Kadokawa and Yoshiro Kaneko
Copyright © 2013 Pan Stanford Publishing Pte. Ltd.
ISBN 978-981-4364-45-4 (Hardcover), ISBN 978-981-4364-46-1 (eBook)
www.panstanford.com

Table 3.1 Characteristics of phosphorylases

EC	Enzyme	Mechanism	Substrate	Product
2.4.1.1	(α-Glucan) phosphorylase	Retention	Glc-α-1,4-Glc	α-Glc-1-P
2.4.1.7	Sucrose phosphorylase	Retention	Glc-α-1,2-Fru	α-Glc-1-P
2.4.1.8	Maltose phosphorylase	Inversion	Glc-α-1,4-Glc	β-Glsc-1-P
2.4.1.20	Cellobiose phosphorylase	Inversion	Glc-β-1,4-Glc	β-Glc-1-P
2.4.1.30	β-1,3-Oligoglucan phosphorylase	Inversion	Glc-β-1,3-Glc	α-Glc-1-P
2.4.1.31	Laminaribiose phosphorylase	Inversion	Glc-β-1,3-Glc	α-Glc-1-P
2.4.1.49	Cellodextrin phosphorylase	Inversion	Glc-β-1,4-Glc	β-Glc-1-P
2.4.1.64	Trehalose phosphorylase	Inversion	Glc-α1,α1-Glc	β-Glc-1-P
2.4.1.97	Laminarin phosphorylase	Inversion	Glc-β-1,3-Glc	α-Glc-1-P
2.4.1.211	β-1,3-Galactosyl-*N*-acetylhexosamine phosphorylase	Inversion	Gal-β-1,3-GlyNAc	α-Gal-1-P
2.4.1.230	Kojibiose phosphorylase	Inversion	Glc-α-1,2-Glc	β-Glc-1-P
2.4.1.231	Trehalose phosphorylase	Retention	Glc-α1,α1-Glc	α-Glc-1-P
—	Chitobiose phosphorylase	Inversion	GlcNAc-β-1,4-GlcNAc	α-GlcNAc-1-P

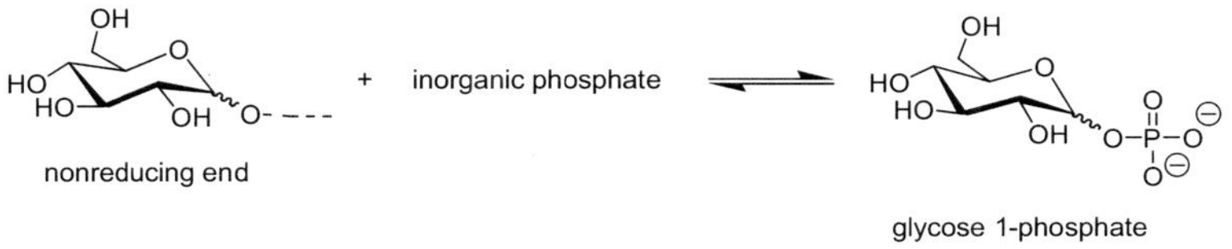

Figure 3.1 Typical phosphorolytic reaction catalyzed by phosphorylase.

to produce the corresponding glycose 1-phosphates and monosaccharides. α-Glucan and cellodextrin phosphorylases have been used in various investigations for the practical synthesis of poly- or oligosaccharides with relatively higher DPs, as well as the related poly- and oligosaccharide-based materials. Although it has been reported that some phosphorylases, such as β-1,3-oligoglucan and kojibiose phosphorylases, recognize glucans with higher DPs and catalyze their phosphorolysis, there have not been many studies on the synthesis of poly- or oligosaccharides catalyzed by these enzymes.

3.2   Outlines of Phosphorylase Catalyses

Of the phosphorylases, α-glucan phosphorylase (glycogen phosphorylase, starch phosphorylase, hereafter, this enzyme is simply called "phosphorylase" in this book) is the most extensively studied and is found in animals, plants, and microorganisms [3]. The role of phosphorylase is considered to be in utilization of storage polysaccharides in the glycolytic pathway. This enzyme catalyzes the reversible phosphorolysis of α-(1→4)-glucans at the nonreducing end, such as glycogen and starch, in the presence of inorganic phosphate, giving rise to α-D-glucose 1-phosphate (Glc-1-P) (Fig. 3.2). The reaction mechanism of phosphorylase is a rapid equilibrium random bi bi mechanism [4]. In animal muscle, phosphorylases are regulated by a phosphorylation/dephosphorylation system comprising a phosphorylase kinase and a phosphorylase phosphatase [5,6]. The phosphororylated and dephosphororylated forms are denoted as phosphorylase *a* and phosphorylase *b*, respectively; the latter has a requirement for adenosine 5′-monophosphate to display activity. In contrast, phosphorylases isolated from plants and microorganisms are not regulated by this system.

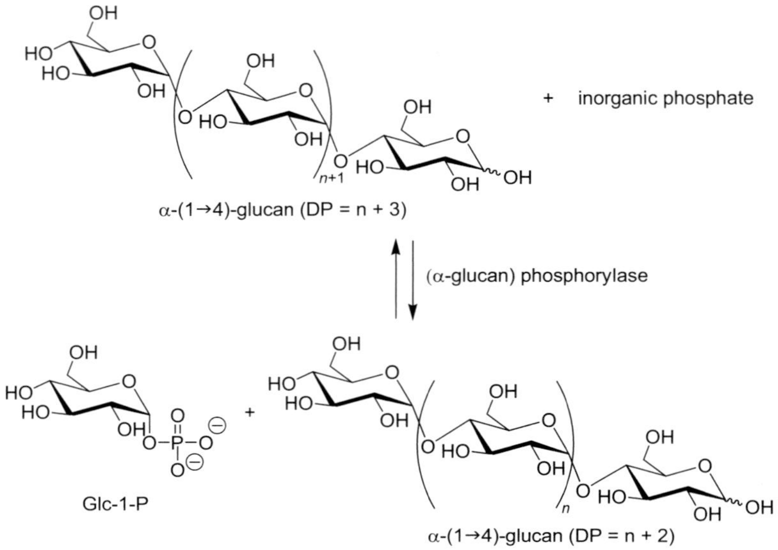

Figure 3.2   Catalysis of phosphorylase.

The second well-studied phosphorylase-type enzyme is sucrose phosphorylase, which catalyzes the reversible phosphorolysis of sucrose into Glc-1-P and fructose in the presence of inorganic phosphate (Fig. 3.3) [7,8]. Therefore, this enzyme has been used with Glc-1-P and fructose for the synthesis of sucrose. Sucrose phosphorylase is found in bacterial cells and is considered to be involved in the metabolism of extracellular sucrose. The phosphorolysis reaction proceeds via a ping-pong bi-bi mechanism and the enzyme transfers α-glucosides even in the absence of inorganic phosphate [9]. Taking into consideration the reaction mechanism, sucrose phosphorylase is an α-glucosyl transferase that also transfers glucose to phosphate [10–12]. This enzyme shows strict substrate specificity with only sucrose, Glc-1-P, and α-D-glucosyl fluoride as a glycosyl donor. However, broad acceptor specificity was found in different studies. Using this enzyme in a transglucosyl manner, several α-glucosides have been synthesized in one step from sucrose and various glycosyl acceptors.

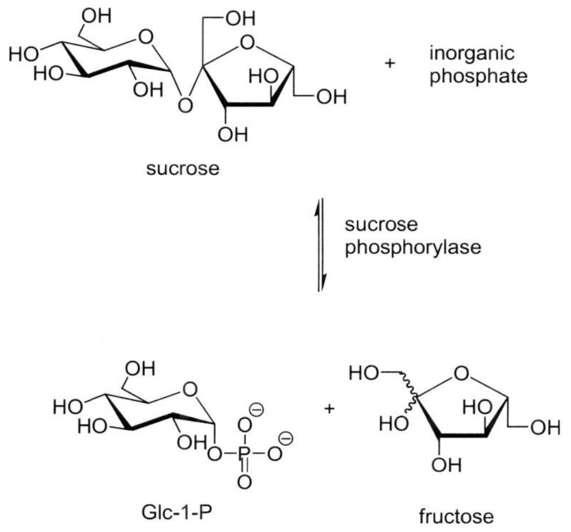

Figure 3.3   Catalysis of sucrose phosphorylase.

Maltose phosphorylase reversibly phosphorolyzes maltose into β-glucose 1-phosphate (β-Glc-1-P) and glucose (Fig. 3.4) [13]. This enzyme has been found in bacterial cells and is considered to be involved in the metabolism of extracellular maltose. Because maltose phosphorylase recognizes the α-anomeric hydroxy group at the reducing end of maltose, it phosphorolyzes only the disaccharide unit.

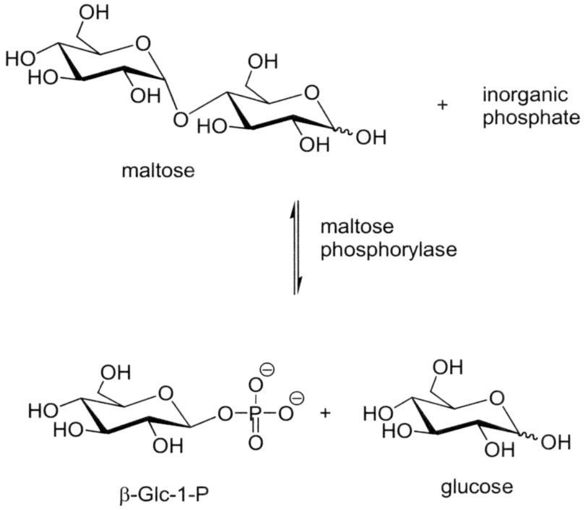

Figure 3.4   Catalysis of maltose phosphorylase.

Cellobiose phosphorylase catalyzes the phosphorolysis of cellobiose with inorganic phosphate by an inversion mechanism to produce Glc-1-P and glucose [14]. This enzyme recognizes the β-anomeric hydroxy group at the reducing end of the cellobiose moiety (Fig. 3.5). Therefore, cellobiose phosphorylase does not phosphorolyze cellooligosaccharide larger than cellobiose. The specificity of acceptor structure in the reverse reaction has also been investigated. Consequently, it was found that this enzyme has a strict specificity for the recognition of the hydroxy groups at positions β-1, 3, and 4 of the glucose but not of the hydroxy groups at positions 2 and 6 [15]. Cellodextrin phosphorylase is an enzyme that catalyzes the reversible phosphorolysis of cellooligosaccharides larger than cellobiose to produce Glc-1-P [16]. The regiospecificity of this enzyme is identical to that of cellobiose phosphorylase, whereas specificity with regard to the DPs of the acceptor is quite different from each other. Therefore, cellooligosaccharides have been synthesized by the cellodextrin phosphorylase-catalyzed chain elongation using various cellobiose acceptors and Glc-1-P donor (Fig. 3.6) [17]. When cellobiose was used as a glycosyl acceptor, various cellooligosaccharides ranging from water-soluble products to crystalline precipitates were obtained, depending on the concentration of the acceptor. The NMR analysis of the crystalline precipitate indicated an average DP of ca. 8. The precipitates showed the diffraction diagrams of low-molecular-weight cellulose II. The cellodextrin phosphorylase-catalyzed synthesis of the cellooligosaccharides substituted at their reducing end was also achieved using various cellobiose derivatives and analogues as a glycosyl acceptor. When the cellodextrin phosphorylase-catalyzed reaction was performed using Glc-1-P as a glycosyl donor and glucose as a glycosyl acceptor, cellooligosaccharides with an average DP of 9 were produced and the products formed highly crystalline cellulose II [18]. Although glucose had been believed to not act as the glycosyl acceptor for the cellodextrin phosphorylase catalysis, a significant amount of insoluble cellulose was precipitated without the accumulation of soluble cellooligosaccharides in this enzymatic reaction system using the glucose acceptor. This result was explained in terms of the large difference in the acceptor reactivity between glucose and cellooligosaccharides as the general acceptor of the cellodextrin phosphorylase catalysis.

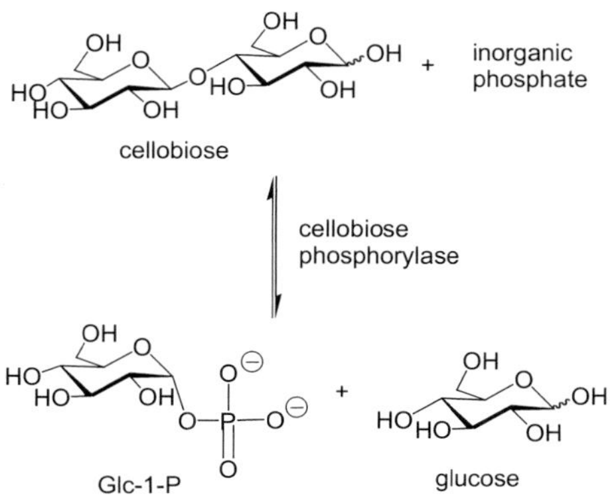

Figure 3.5 Catalysis of cellobiose phosphorylase.

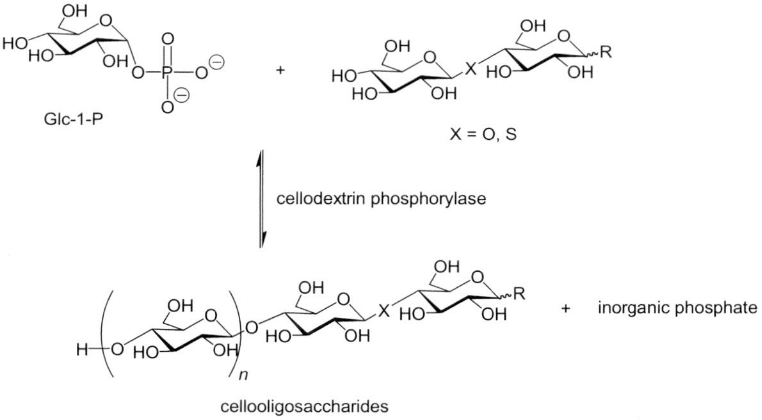

Figure 3.6 Cellodextrin phosphorylase-catalyzed synthesis of cellooligosaccharides.

Cellodextrin phosphorylase was found to recognize α-D-xylose 1-phosphate (Xyl-1-P) as a glycosyl donor and xylose-containing disaccharides as a glycosyl acceptor [19]. Therefore, the enzymatic synthesis of a library of β-(1→4)-hetero-glucose and xylose-based oligosaccharides was attempted by the cellodextrin phosphorylase-catalyzed glycosylation using Glc-1-P or Xyl-1-P as a donor and cellobiose, xylobiose, Glc-β-(1→4)-Xyl, or Xyl-β-(1→4)-Glc as an acceptor (Fig. 3.7). Consequently, the enzymatic glycosylation by the cellodextrin phosphorylase catalysis produced all six

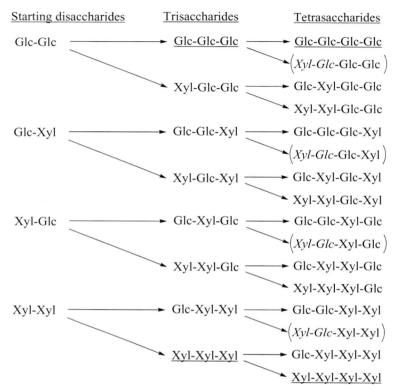

Figure 3.7 Synthesis of a library of β-(1→4)-hetero-glucose and xylose-based oligosaccharides by the cellodextrin phosphorylase-catalyzed glycosylation (except underlined cello- and xylooligosaccharides); the four tetrasaccharides in parentheses were not obtained successfully.

heterotrisaccharides and 10 of 14 possible heterotetrasaccharides. However, it was found that it is not possible to synthesize the four tetrasaccharides with a Xyl→Glc sequence at their nonreducing ends (in parentheses in Fig. 3.7) by this enzymatic reaction.

Two enzymes exist for the phosphorolysis of trehalose: inversion type (EC 2.4.1.64) and retention type (EC 2.4.1.231) [20,21]. The former reversibly phosphorolyzes trehalose to form β-Glc-1-P and glucose and the latter catalyzes the same reaction but with a retention of the anomeric configuration, giving Glc-1-P and glucose (Fig. 3.8). In an interesting application, a process is described for producing

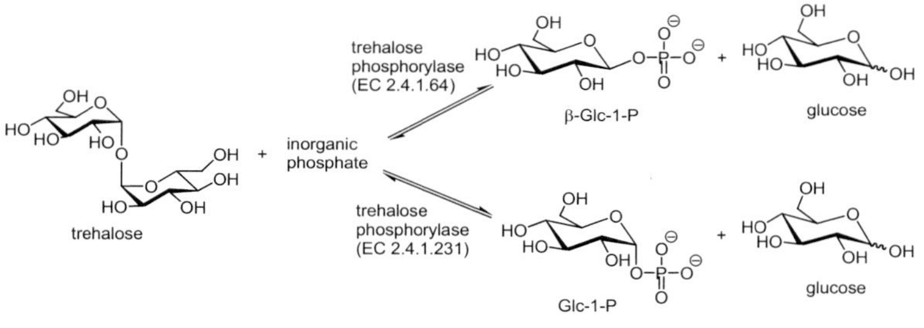

Figure 3.8 Catalyses of trehalose phosphorylases.

trehalose where maltose phosphorylase and the inversion type trehalose phosphorylase act on maltose in the presence of inorganic phosphate [22]. In principle, it should also be possible to use sucrose phosphorylase and the retaining type trehalose phosphorylase acting on sucrose in the presence of inorganic phosphate.

Kojibiose phosphorylase was found in the cell-free extract of a thermophilic bacterium accompanied with trehalose phosphorylase [23]. This enzyme catalyzes the reversible phosphorolysis of kojibiose into β-Glc-1-P and glucose. The reverse reaction by kojibiose phosphorylase catalysis was utilized for the synthesis of kojioligosaccharides (Fig. 3.9) [24]. When the mixtures of various proportions of glucose and β-Glc-1-P were allowed to react in the presence of kojibiose phosphorylase, kojioligosaccharides were produced. The average DPs of the products increased with the decreasing proportions of glucose.

Three enzymes catalyze the phosphorolysis of β-(1→3)-linked glucans: β-1,3-oligoglucan phosphorylase (EC 2.4.1.30), laminaribiose phosphorylase (EC 2.4.1.31), and laminarin

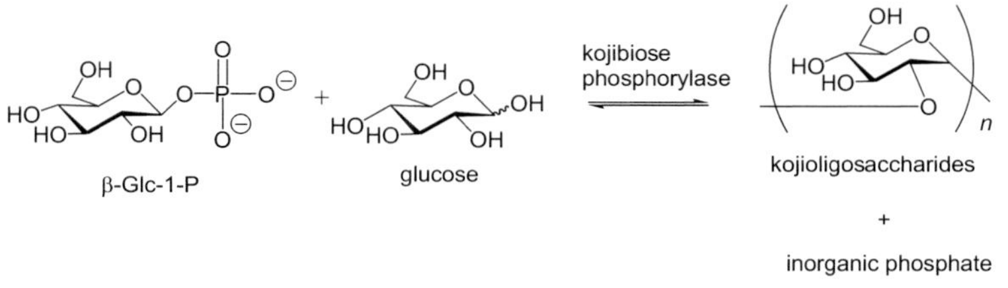

Figure 3.9 Kojibiose phosphorylase-catalyzed synthesis of kojioligosaccharides.

phosphorylase (EC 2.4.1.97) [25–27]. These three enzymes have been found as intracellular enzymes in algae and euglenida cells. β-1,3-Oligoglucan and laminaribiose phosphorylases are found in *Euglea gracilis* and catalyze the reversible phosphorolysis of laminaribiose and its trimer, and also higher oligomers. Inversion of the anomeric configuration occurs with these enzymes, giving rise to Glc-1-P. The key difference in the reactions catalyzed by these two enzymes is that β-1,3-oligoglucan phosphorylase phosphorolyzes laminaritriose faster than lamianribiose and vise versa for lamiaribiose phosphorylase. A mixture of laminarioligosaccharides with varying DPs was synthesized from glucose and Glc-1-P by the combined actions of these two enzymes [28]. In contrast to these two enzymes, laminarin phosphorylase phosphorolyzes a polymeric substrate.

β-1,3-Galactosyl-*N*-acetylhexosamine phosphorylase catalyzes the phosphorolysis of Gal-β-(1→3)-GlcNAc or Gal-β-(1→3)-GalNAc oligosaccharides [30]. In the reverse reaction, this enzyme specifically recognizes α-galactose 1-phosphate as a donor and GlcNAc and GalNAc as acceptors. Chitobiose phosphorylase phosphorolyzes the conversion of *N,N′*-diacetylchitobiose into α-GlcNAc 1-phosphate and GlcNAc [30].

3.3   Phosphorylase-Catalyzed Glycosylation

As mentioned earlier, phosphorylase catalyzes the reversible phosphorolytic reaction of α-(1→4)-glucans at the nonreducing end in the presence of inorganic phosphate, giving Glc-1-P (Fig. 3.2) [1]. By means of reversibility of the reaction, α-(1→4)-glycosidic linkage can be constructed by the phosphorylase-catalyzed glycosylation using Glc-1-P as a glycosyl donor [31]. As a glycosyl acceptor in the glycosylation reaction, maltooligosaccharides with DPs higher than the smallest one, which is recognized by phosphorylase, are used. The glycosyl acceptor is often called a "primer." The smallest glycosyl acceptor for the phosphorylase-catalyzed glycosylation is typically maltotetraose (Glc_4), whereas that for the phosphorolysis is maltopentaose (Glc_5). In the glycosylation, a glucose unit is transferred from Glc-1-P to a nonreducing end of the primer to form α-(1→4)-glycosidic linkage. When the excess molar ratio of Glc-

1-P to the primer is present in the reaction mixture, the successive glycosylations occur as a propagation of polymerization to produce the α-(1→4)-glucan chain, i.e., amylose.

Because phosphorylase has shown loose specificity for the recognition of the structure of the glycosyl donor, the phosphorylase-catalyzed glycosylation using different glycose 1-phosphates has been performed to produce nonnatural oligosaccharides. For example, the enzymatic synthesis of α-D-xylosylated maltooligosaccharides by the phosphorylase-catalyzed α-xylosylation using Xyl-1-P was reported (Fig. 3.10) [32]. Because the structural difference of Xyl-1-P from Glc-1-P was only the absence of a CH_2OH group at position 6, a high possibility for recognition of this nonnative substrate by phosphorylase had been supposed. When the phosphorylase-catalyzed enzymatic reaction using Xyl-1-P as a glycosyl donor and Glc_4 as a glycosyl acceptor was carried out, xylosylated oligosaccharides were produced, which was confirmed by the MALDI-TOF MS and ^1H NMR spectra of the crude products. Furthermore, the MALDI-TOF MS spectrum showed small peaks assignable to the oligosaccharides consisting of two xylose units in addition to the main peaks ascribable to the oligosaccharide having one xylose unit. However, the aforementioned analytical data did not provide sufficient evidence to determine the structures of the products, in

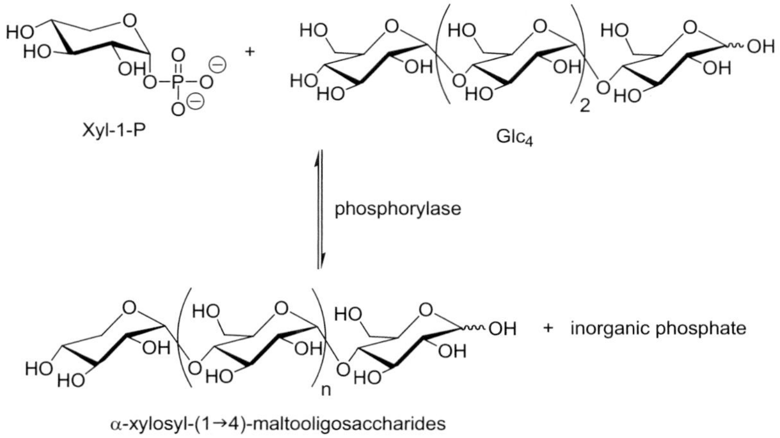

Figure 3.10 Phosphorylase-catalyzed α-xylosylation of Glc_4 using Xyl-1-P.

which the xylose unit was positioned at the nonreducing end of the xylosylated oligosaccharides. Consequently, the treatment of the reaction mixture with glucoamylase (GA, EC 3.2.1.3), which catalyzed an exo-wise hydrolysis at the nonreducing end of α-$(1{\rightarrow}4)$-glucans, to reveal whether the xylose unit was positioned at the nonreducing end. If the xylose unit is positioned at the nonreducing end of a maltooligosaccharide, GA does not recognize it as a substrate. The ^{1}H NMR spectrum of the treated products indicated the remaining signals due to the xylosidic linkages, supporting that the xylose unit was positioned at the nonreducing end. Furthermore, the main product was isolated from the crude mixture using high performance liquid chromatography (HPLC) and the structure was confirmed by the ^{1}H NMR spectrum to be α-D-xylosyl-$(1{\rightarrow}4)$-Glc$_4$. For further analysis, the formation of the xylosylated maltooligosaccharides vs. reaction time in the phosphorylase-catalyzed α-xylosylation was evaluated under the conditions as the feed molar ratios of Glc$_4$ to Xyl-1-P as 1:10, 1:5, and 1:1. The total yields of the xylosylated products were estimated by the integrated ratios in the ^{1}H NMR spectra of the crude products. Highest yields of 44% (1:10), 25% (1:5), and 10% (1:1) based on the amounts of Glc$_4$ used were obtained after 48 h. Schwarz *et al.* reported the kinetic analysis using Glc-1-P and Xyl-1-P in the phosphorylase-catalyzed reaction. Phosphorylase displayed a very large kinetic selectivity ratio, i.e., $k_{\text{catGlc-1-P}}/k_{\text{catXyl-1-P}}$ = 2000 [33].

The phosphorylase-catalyzed α-mannosylation using α-mannose 1-phosphate (Man-1-P) was also examined (Fig. 3.11) [34]. Although the equatorial hydroxy group is not essential for phosphorylase, 2-epimer of Glc-1-P, i.e., Man-1-P, is expected to have a low affinity to the enzyme owing to steric hindrance by the axial hydroxy group. In the crude products obtained by the phosphorylase-catalyzed reaction of Man-1-P with Glc$_4$, mannosylated compounds were found. A pentasaccharide fraction was isolated by size exclusion chromatography and the structures were confirmed by the ^{1}H NMR spectrum to be a mixture of Glc$_5$ and α-mannosyl-$(1{\rightarrow}4)$-Glc$_4$. The mixture was not separated completely. Particularly, the position of the mannose unit was assigned owing to the lower intensity of the terminal H-4 signal in comparison with the integral of α- and β-H-1 at the reducing end.

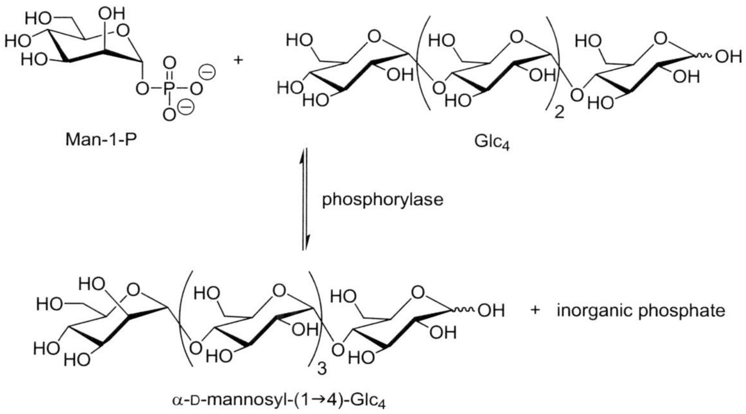

α-D-mannosyl-(1→4)-Glc₄

Figure 3.11 Phosphorylase-catalyzed α-mannosylation of Glc₄ using Man-1-P.

Withers *et al.* enzymatically prepared 2-deoxy-α-glucose 1-phosphate (dGlc-1-P) in a two-step process (Fig. 3.12) [35]. First, a 2-deoxyglucose unit is transferred to the α-glucan primer that is catalyzed by inorganic phosphate. In the second step, 2-deoxyglucose is released by phosphorolysis to produce dGlc-1-P and in the overall reaction the primer remains unchanged. On the basis of this study, 1,2-dideoxyglucose (glucal) was applied as a glycosyl donor in considerable excess in order to shift the equilibrium to the chain elongation with a glucal to primer ratio of 15:1 for the occurrence of 2-deoxyglucosylation in the presence of inorganic phosphate (Fig. 3.13) [36]. After the phosphorylase-catalyzed reaction in the presence of glucal, Glc₄, and only 0.05 equiv. of phosphate for 6 h, 2-deoxy-α-glucosylated penta-, hexa-, and heptasaccharides were separated by size exclusion chromatography in 17%, 12%, and 8% yields, respectively. Additionally, a fraction of higher molecular weight with an average DP of 12 was obtained in 33% yield.

Withers also reported the phosphorylase-catalyzed glycosylation of glycogen with 3- or 4-deoxy-α-glucose 1-phosphates. However, only averages of up to 1.5 units were transferred [37].

Oligosaccharides containing GlcN units and its derivatives, e.g., GlcNAc, serve key functions for living organisms such as in cell–cell recognition and immune responses. The preparation of saccharide chains containing GlcN residues, therefore, has been frequently required for the various studies in glycoscience. Much effort has

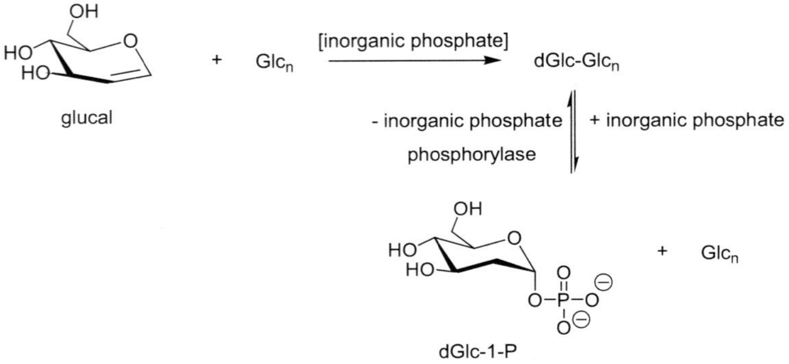

Figure 3.12 Two-step synthesis of dGlc-1-P in the presence of inorganic phosphate and phosphorylase.

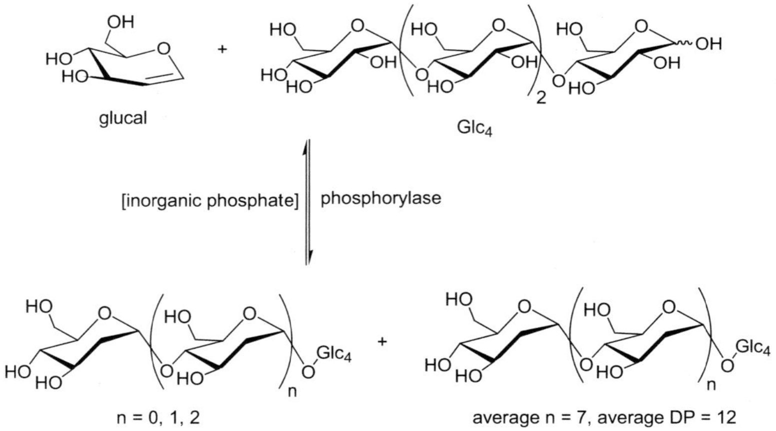

Figure 3.13 Phosphorylase-catalyzed synthesis of 2-deoxy-α-glucosylated oligosaccharides.

been focused on glycosylation using glycosyl donors derived from GlcNAc and other *N*-substituted GlcN residues, such as oxazoline glycosylation [38,39]. However, the glycosylation of a GlcN donor with a free amino group had hardly been achieved. On the basis of these viewpoints, it was reported that GlcN-1-P was recognized as the glycosyl donor in the phosphorylase-catalyzed glycosylation to form α-(1→4)-glucosaminyl linkage [40]. This was the first example of the enzymatic α-glucosaminylation using the GlcN donor with a free amino group.

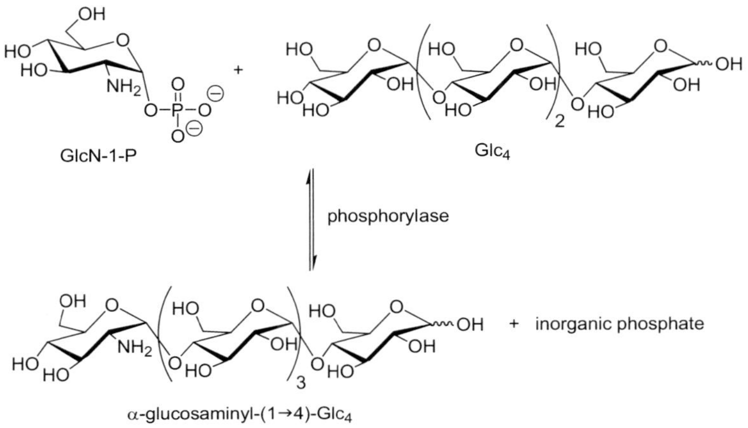

Figure 3.14 Phosphorylase-catalyzed α-glucosaminylation of Glc$_4$ using GlcN-1-P.

The phosphorylase-catalyzed α-glucosaminylation was performed using GlcN-1-P as a glycosyl donor and Glc$_4$ as a glycosyl acceptor (Fig. 3.13). After the reaction mixture was lyophilized, *N*-acetylation was carried out using acetic anhydride, and the transfer of a GlcN unit to the primer was evaluated by MALDI-TOF MS measurement. Because the difference in the molecular masses of the anhydroglucose and anhydroglucosamine units was only 1, which could be made larger by the *N*-acetylation of the latter unit, the measurement was performed on the *N*-acetylated material. In the MALDI-TOF MS spectrum of the *N*-acetylated crude products, a significant peak corresponding to the mass of a pentasaccharide containing one GlcNAc unit was observed. This data indicated that one GlcN residue transferred from GlcN-1-P to Glc$_4$ by the phosphorylase-catalyzed α-glucosaminylation. To confirm the presence of the GlcN unit at a nonreducing end of the produced oligosaccharide, the treatment of the *N*-acetylated crude products with GA was performed. In the MALDI-TOF MS spectrum of the treated product, the peak assigned to the molecular mass of the *N*-acetylgucosaminylated Glc$_4$ remained intact, supporting that the GlcNAc unit was positioned at the nonreducing end. If the transfer of one GlcN residue from Glc-1-P to Glc$_4$ proceeded once, further glucosaminylation was probably suppressed because the glucosaminylated Glc$_4$ was not recognized as the acceptor by phosphorylase. The main product was isolated from the *N*-acetylated crude mixture after the treatment with GA using HPLC. The ^{1}H NMR spectrum of the isolated material fully supported the structure of *N*-acetyl-α-glucosaminyl-$(1\rightarrow4)$-Glc$_4$. In particular, there was no signal assigned to the H-4 position of the glucose residue at the nonreducing end of Glc$_4$, whereas the signal ascribed to the free H-4 position of GlcNAc was observed. This observation indicated that the GlcNAc unit was positioned at the nonreducing end bound with the α-$(1\rightarrow4)$-glycosidic linkage.

Although the phosphorylase-catalyzed glycosylation of Glc$_4$ using GlcNAc-1-P as a glycosyl donor was also performed under the same conditions as those using GlcN-1-P, the MALDL-TOF MS spectrum of the crude products did not show peaks assignable to the molecular masses of oligosaccharides having a GlcNAc unit. This result indicated that the GlcNAc-1-P was not recognized by phosphorylase, probably because the bulky acetamido group in GlcNAc-1-P blocked approach to the active site.

However, the following study reported that 2-deoxy-2-formamido-α-glucosamine 1-phosphate (GlcNF-1-P), which had the formamido group of a smaller substituent than an acetamido, was recognized as a glycosyl donor by phosphorylase [41]. This allowed the *N*-formyl-α-glucosaminylation of maltooligosaccharide to give *N*-formyl-α-glucosaminylated maltooligosaccharides (Fig. 3.15). The MALDI-TOF MS spectrum of the crude products obtained by the phosphorylase-catalyzed *N*-formyl-α-glucosaminylation using GlcNF-1-P and Glc$_4$ showed only a significant peak corresponding to the mass of a pentasaccharide containing one GlcNF unit. This data indicated that the transfer of one GlcNF residue from GlcNF-1-P to Glc$_4$ occurred. Then, the treatment of the crude products with GA was carried out to reveal whether the GlcNF unit was positioned at the nonreducing end. In the MALDI-TOF MS spectrum of the treated products, the peak assigned to the molecular mass of the produced pentasaccharide remained intact, supporting that the GlcNF unit was positioned at the nonreducing end. Moreover, the pentasaccharide was isolated from the crude products after the treatment with GA. The ^{1}H NMR spectrum of the isolated material fully supported the structure of *N*-formyl-α-glucosaminyl-$(1\rightarrow4)$-Glc$_4$. The two signals due to the formyl group were observed, which were assignable to *E*- and *Z*-isomers owing to hindered rotation of the formyl C–N bond (two rotamers). For further analysis, the formation of *N*-formyl-α-glucosaminylated oligosaccharides vs. reaction time

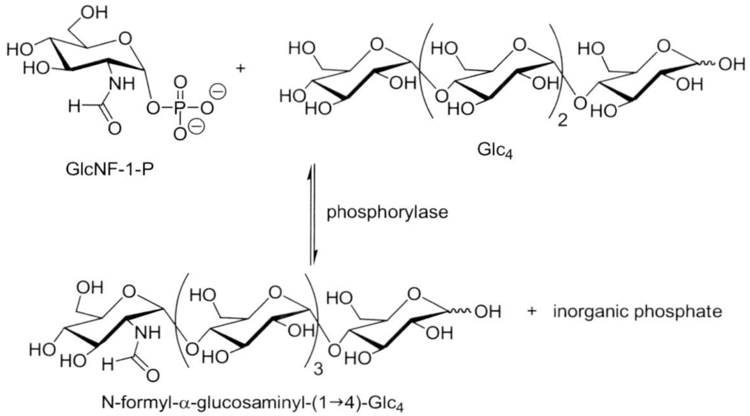

Figure 3.15 Phosphorylase-catalyzed *N*-formyl-α-glucosaminylation of Glc$_4$ using GlcNF-1-P.

in the phosphorylase-catalyzed glycosylation using GlcNF-1-P and Glc$_4$ (5:1) was evaluated and compared with that using GlcN-1-P as well as Glc-1-P under the same conditions. The total yields of the glycosylated products were calculated on the basis of the amounts of inorganic phosphate produced from the glycose 1-phosphates by the phosphorylase catalysis. A reaction time of 4 days in the glycosylation using GlcNF-1-P gave 33% yield of the products based on the amount of Glc$_4$, whereas the yield was 72% in the glycosylation using GlcN-1-P. These data indicated that the phosphorylase recognized GlcN-1-P more efficiently than GlcNF-1-P. However, the reaction using Glc-1-P was much faster than such two reactions and yield reached almost 100% in 45 min, because Glc-1-P is the native substrate for phosphorylase catalysis.

The phosphorylase-catalyzed *N*-formyl-α-glucosaminylation using GlcNF-1-P was also conducted in the presence of Glc$_3$ or Glc$_5$. In the MALDI-TOF MS spectrum of the crude products using Glc$_3$, no peaks assignable to the molecular masses of oligosaccharides having a GlcNF unit were observed, indicating no occurrence of *N*-formyl-α-glucosaminylation of Glc$_3$ by GlcNF-1-P. Because the smallest glycosyl acceptor for the phosphorylase-catalyzed glycosylation was Glc$_4$, Glc$_3$ was not recognized by phosphorylase. In the MALDI-TOF MS spectrum of the crude products using Glc$_5$, however, several peaks separated by m/z equal to 162 were observed, which correspond to

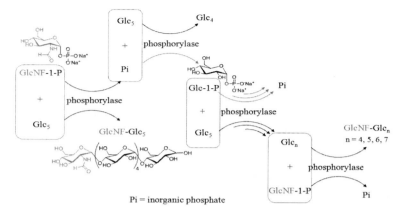

Figure 3.16 Plausible pathway in phosphorylase-catalyzed N-formyl-α-glucosaminylation of Glc$_5$.

the molecular masses of pentasaccharide–octasaccharide containing a GlcNF unit. This finding indicated the occurrence of both the N-formyl-α-glucosaminylation by GlcNF-1-P and α-glucosylation by Glc-1-P when Glc$_5$ was used as a glycosyl acceptor (Fig. 3.16). Because Glc$_5$ is the smallest substrate for phosphorolysis in the presence of inorganic phosphate, Glc-1-P was possibly produced by phosphorolysis of Glc$_5$ with simultaneous production of Glc$_4$ at the early stage of the reaction, where inorganic phosphate was formed by the transfer of a GlcNF unit from GlcNF-1-P to Glc$_5$. Then, Glc-1-P was recognized more efficiently by phosphorylase than GlcNF-1-P. Thus, the maltooligosaccharides with larger DPs, such as Glc$_6$ and Glc$_7$, were produced by the transfer of the glucose residue from Glc-1-P to Glc$_4$ or Glc$_5$. Furthermore, if N-formyl-α-glucosaminylation of the produced maltooligosaccharides by GlcNF-1-P proceeded once, subsequent glycosylation was suppressed because the N-formyl-α-glucosaminylated oligosaccharides were less efficiently recognized by phosphorylase.

References

1. Kitaoka, M., and Hayashi, K. (2002). Carbohydrate-processing phosphorolytic enzymes, *Trends Glycosci. Glycotechnol.*, **14**, pp. 35–50.

2. Seibel, J., Jördening, H.-J., and Buchholz, K. (2006). Glycosylation with activated sugars using glycosyltransferases and transglycosidases, *Biocatal. Biotranform.*, **24**, pp. 311–342.

3. Fletterick, R. J., and Sprang, S. R. (1982). Glycogen phosphorylase structures and function, *Acc. Chem. Res.*, **15**, pp. 361–369.

4. Gold, A. M., Johnson, R. M., and Sánchez, G. R. (1971). Kinetic mechanism of potato phosphorylase, *J. Biol. Chem.*, **246**, pp. 3444–3450.

5. Krebs, E. G., and Fischer, E. H. (1956). The phosphorylase *b* to *a* converting enzyme of rabbit skeletal muscle, *Biochim. Biophys. Acta*, **20**, pp. 150–157.

6. Graves, D. J., Fischer, E. H., and Krebs, E. G. (1960). Specificity studies on muscle phosphorylase phosphatase, *J. Biol. Chem.*, **235**, pp. 805–809.

7. Doudoroff, M. (1941). Studies on the phosphorolysis of sucrose, *J. Biol. Chem.*, **151**, pp. 351–361.

8. Taylor, F., Chen, L., Gong, C. S., and Tsao, G. T. (1982). Kinetics of immobilized sucrose phosphorylase, *Biotechnol. Bioeng.*, **24**, pp. 317–328.

9. Silverstein, R., Voet, J., Reed, D., and Abeles, R. H. (1967). Purification and mechanism of action of sucrose phosphorylase, *J. Biol. Chem.*, **242**, pp. 1338–1346.

10. Kitao, S., and Sekine, H. (1992). Transglucosylation catalyzed by sucrose phosphorylase from leuconostoc mesenteroides and production of glucosyl-xylitol, *Biosci. Biotechnol. Biochem.*, **56**, pp. 2011–2014.

11. Kitao, S., Ariga, T., Matsudo, T., and Sekine, H. (1993). The syntheses of catechin-glucosides by transglycosylation with leuconostoc mesenteroides sucrose phosphorylase, *Biosci. Biotechnol. Biochem.*, **57**, pp. 2010–2015.

12. Kitao, S., and Sekine, H. (1994). α-D-Glucosyl transfer to phenolic compounds by sucrose phosphorylase from leuconostoc mesenteroides and production of α-arbutin, *Biosci. Biotechnol. Biochem.*, **58**, pp. 38–42.

13. Fitting, C., and Doudoroff, M. (1952). Phosphorolysis of maltose by enzyme preparations from neisseria meningitidis, *J. Biol. Chem.*, **199**, pp. 153–163.

14. Ayers, W. A. (1959). Phosphorolysis and synthesis of cellobiose by cell extracts from *Ruminococcus flavefaciens*, *J. Biol. Chem.*, **234**, pp. 2819–2822.

15. Kitaoka, M., Sasaki, T., and Taniguchi, H. (1992). Synthetic reaction of cellvibrio-gilvus cellobiose phosphorylase, *J. Biochem.*, **112**, pp. 40–44.

16. Sheth, K., and Alexander, J. K. (1969). Purification and properties of β-1,4-oligoglucan: Orthophosphate glucosyltransferase from *Clostridium thermocellum*, *J. Biol. Chem.*, **244**, pp. 457–464.

17. Samain, E., Lancelon-Pin, C., FéRigo, F., Moreau, V., Chanzy, H., Heyraud, A., and Driguez, H. (1995). Phosphorolytic synthesis of cellodextrins, *Carbohydr. Res.*, **271**, pp. 217–226.

18. Hiraishi, M., Igarashi, K., Kimura, S., Wada, M., and Kitaoka, M. (2009). Synthesis of highly ordered cellulose II *in vitro* using cellodextrin phosphorylase, *Carbohydr. Res.*, **344**, pp. 2468–2473.

19. Shintate, K., Kitaoka, M., Kim, Y.-K., and Hayashi, K. (2003). Enzymatic synthesis of a library of β-(1→4) hetero-D-glucose and D-xylose-based oligosaccharides employing cellodextrin phosphorylase, *Carbohydr. Res.*, **338**, pp. 1981–1990.

20. Maréchal, L. R., and Belocopitow, E. (1972). Metabolism of Trehalose in *Euglena gracilis*: I. Partial purification and some properties of trehalose phosphorylase, *J. Biol. Chem.*, **247**, pp. 3223–3228.

21. Kitamoto, Y., Akashi, H., Tanaka, H., and Mori, N. (1988). α-Glucose-1-phosphate formation by a novel trehalose phosphorylase from *Flammulina velutipes*, *FEMS Microbiol. Lett.*, **55**, pp. 147–150.

22. Murao, S., Nagano, H., Ogura, S., and Nishino, T. (1985). Enzymatic synthesis of trehalose from maltose, *Agri. Biol. Chem.*, **49**, pp. 2113–2118.

23. Chaen, H., Yamamoto, T., Nishimoto, T., Nakada, T., Fukuda, S., Sugimoto, T., Kurimoto, M., and Tsujisaka, Y. (1999). Purification and characterization of a novel phosphorylase, kojibiose phosphorylase, from *Thermoanaerobium brockii*, *J. Appl. Glycosci.*, **46**, pp. 423–429.

24. Chaen, H., Nishimoto, T., Nakada, T., Fukuda, S., Kurimoto, M., and Tsujisaka, Y. (2001). Enzymatic synthesis of kojioligosaccharides using kojibiose phosphorylase, *J. Biosci. Bioeng.*, **92**, pp. 177–182.

25. Goldemberg, S. H., Maréchal, L. R., and De Souza, B. C. (1966). β-1,3-Oligoglucan: Orthophosphate glucosyltransferase from *Euglena gracilis*, *J. Biol. Chem.*, **241**, pp. 45–50.

26. Maréchal, L. R. (1967). β-1,3-Oligoglucan: Orthophosphate glucosyltransferases from *Euglena gracilis*: I. Isolation and some properties of a β-1,3-oligoglucan phosphorylase, *Biochim. Biophys. Acta Enzymol.*, **146**, pp. 417–430.

27. Albrecht, G. J., and Kauss, H. (1971). Purification, crystallization and properties of a β-(1→3)-glucan phosphorylase from *Ochromonas malhamensis*, *Phytochemistry*, **10**, pp. 1293–1298.

28. Kitaoka, M., Sasaki, T., and Taniguchi, H. (1991). Synthesis of laminarioligosaccharides using crude extract of *Euglena gracilis* z cells, *Agric. Biol. Chem.*, **55**, pp. 1431–1432.

29. Derensy-Dron, D., Krzewinski, F., Brassart, C., and Boucuelet, S. (1999). β-1,2-Galactosyl-*N*-acetylhexosamine phosphorylase from *Bifidobacterium bifidum* DSM 20082: Characterization, partial purification and relation to mucin degradation, *Biotechnol. Appl. Biochem.*, **29**, pp. 3–10.

30. Park, J. K., Keyhani, N. O., and Roseman, S. (2000). Chitin catabolism in the marine bacterium *Vibrio furnissii:* Identification, molecular cloning, and characterization of a *N,N´*-diacetylchitobiose phosphorylse, *J. Biol. Chem.*, **275**, pp. 33077–33083.

31. Ziegast, G., and Pfannemüller, B. (1987). Phosphorolytic syntheses with di-, oligo- and multi-functional primers, *Carbohydr. Res.*, **160**, pp. 185–204.

32. Nawaji, M., Izawa, H., Kaneko, Y., and Kadokawa, J. (2008). Enzymatic synthesis of α-D-xylosylated maltooligosaccharides by phosphorylase-catalyzed xylosylation, *J. Carbohydr. Chem.*, **27**, pp. 214–222.

33. Schwarz, A., Pierfederici, F. M., and Nidetzky, B. (2005). Catalytic mechanism of α-retaining glucosyl transfer by *Corynebacterium callunase* starch phosphorylase: The role of histidine-334 examined through kinetic characterization of site-directed mutants, *Biochem. J.*, **387**, pp. 437–445.

34. Evers, B., and Thiem, J. (1997). Further syntheses employing phosphorylase, *Bioorg. Med. Chem.*, **5**, pp. 857–863.

35. Percival, M. D., and Withers, S. G. (1988). Application of enzymes in the synthesis and hydrolytic study of 2-deoxy-α-D-glucopyranosyl phosphate, *Can. J. Chem.*, **66**, pp. 1970–1972.

36. Evers, B., Mischnick, P., and Thiem, J. (1994). Synthesis of 2-deoxy-α-D-*arabino*-hexopyranosyl phosphate and 2-deoxy-maltooligosaccharides with phosphorylase, *Carbohydr. Res.*, **262**, pp. 335–341.

37. Withers, S. G. (1990). The enzymic synthesis and NMR characterization of specifically deoxygenated and fluorinated glycogens, *Carbohydr. Res.*, **197**, pp. 61–73.

38. Kobayashi, S., Ohmae, M., Fujikawa, S., and Ochiai, H. (2005). Enzymatic precision polymerization for synthesis of glycosaminoglycans and their derivatives, *Macromol. Symp.*, **226**, pp. 147–156.

39. Ohmae, M., Fujikawa, S., Ochiai, H., and Kobayashi S. (2006). Enzyme-catalyzed synthesis of natural and unnatural polysaccharides, *J. Polym. Sci., Part A: Polym. Chem.*, **44**, pp. 5014–5027.

40. Nawaji, M., Izawa, H., Kaneko, Y., and Kadokawa, J. (2008). Enzymatic α-glucosaminylation of maltooligosaccharides catalyzed by phosphorylase, *Carbohydr. Res.*, **343**, pp. 2692–2696.

41. Kawazoe, S., Izawa, H., Nawaji, M., Kaneko, Y., and Kadokawa, J. (2010). Phosphorylase-catalyzed *N*-formyl-α-glucosaminylation of maltooligosaccharides, *Carbohydr. Res.*, **345**, pp. 631–636.

Chapter 4

Phosphorylase-Catalyzed Enzymatic Polymerization

4.1 Outlines of Phosphorylase-Catalyzed Polymerization

Amylose is expected to have uses in various industries as a functional biomaterial. Amylose is one of the components of starch and present with amylopectin in nature (Chapter 1). However, pure amylose is currently not available for industrial purposes because the separation of natural amylose from amylopectin is difficult. Phosphorylase is the only enzyme that can produce amylose with the desired average molecular weight (Fig. 4.1) [1]. Phosphorylases from potato and rabbit muscle have been successfully employed in the synthesis of amylose *in vitro* [2,3]. As a glycosyl acceptor for the initiation of the polymerization, maltooligosaccharides with DPs higher than the smallest one, i.e., maltotetraose, which is recognized by phosphorylase, are used. The glycosyl acceptor is often called a "primer." In the initiation, a glucose unit is transferred from Glc-1-P of a monomer to a nonreducing end of the primer to form α-(1→4)-glycosidic linkage. Then, successive reactions in the same manner occur as a propagation of the polymerization to produce the α-(1→4)-glucan chain, i.e., amylose. Because the phosphorylase-catalyzed polymerization proceeds analogously to a living polymerization, the

Engineering of Polysaccharide Materials: By Phosphorylase-Catalyzed Enzymatic Chain-Elongation
Jun-ichi Kadokawa and Yoshiro Kaneko
Copyright © 2013 Pan Stanford Publishing Pte. Ltd.
ISBN 978-981-4364-45-4 (Hardcover), ISBN 978-981-4364-46-1 (eBook)
www.panstanford.com

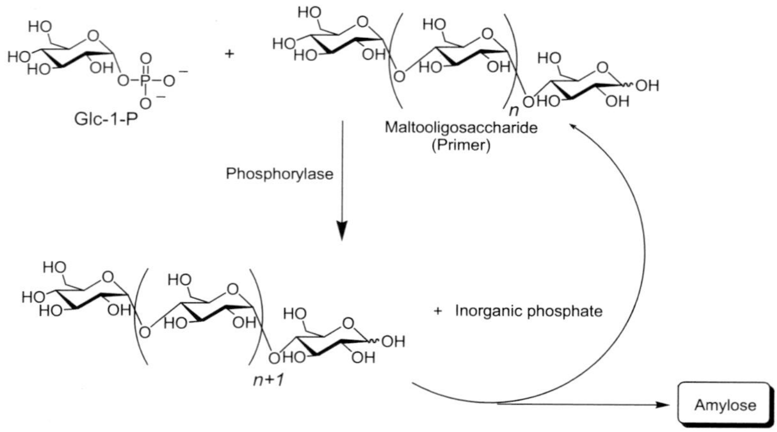

Figure 4.1 Phosphorylase-catalyzed enzymatic polymerization to amylose.

molecular weight of the produced amylose has a narrow distribution ($M_w/M_n < 1.2$) and can be controlled by the Glc-1-P/primer feed molar ratios [4].

It has been reported that phosphorylase from rabbit muscle is more suitable for the synthesis of amylose with low molecular weight in DPs ranging 10–20 than that from potato [3].

4.2 Thermostable Phosphorylase Catalysis

The phosphorylase from potato has been studied extensively and is known to elongate the α-glucan chain rapidly by using maltotetraose as a primer. However, the potato phosphorylase is not suitable for industrial processes because of its low thermostability. Amylose is known to precipitate at low temperatures, but this can be significantly inhibited at elevated temperatures. Thermostable phosphorylases have been employed for the enzymatic synthesis of amylose at elevated temperatures. The phosphorylase genes from several thermophilic microorganisms such as *Bacillus stearothermophilus* [4], *Thermus thermophilus* [5], *Thermococcus litoralis* [6], and *Thermus aquaticus* [7] have been isolated.

Phosphorylase from *T. aquaticus* showed extensive thermal stability where the enzyme retained 80% of its activity even after incubation at 80°C for 30 min [7]. Incubation of the *T. aquaticus* phosphorylase with various Glc-1-P/primer ratios at 70°C resulted in synthesis of amylose with a distinct molecular weight. The M_w/M_n value of each amylose was almost 1, indicating the product had very narrow molecular weight distribution. This narrow distribution might reflect the fact that amylose does not form a precipitate at this high reaction temperature. In this case, however, the maximum M_w of the product was 1.24×10^5 and the yield of amylose decreased as the Glc-1-P/primer ratio increased.

It has been reported that the smallest primer for the glucan synthesis reaction of potato phosphorylase is maltotetraose, and the smallest substrate for the phosphorolysis was maltopentaose. However, phosphorylase from *T. aquaticus* shows distinct substrate specificity, where maltotriose is the smallest primer for glucan synthesis and the maltotetraose is the smallest substrate for phosphorolysis [7]. This unique substrate specificity is also an advantage for the production of amylose because a cheaper primer can be used.

4.3 Practical Applications of Phosphorylase-Catalyzed Polymerization

Apparent production of an enzymatically synthesized amylose in DMSO was carried out by means of the calcium alginate hydrogel beads/DMSO system as the reaction field of the phosphorylase-catalyzed polymerization (Fig. 4.2) [8]. When the calcium alginate hydrogel beads including Glc-1-P, maltoheptaose, and phosphorylase were suspended in DMSO and the system was slowly stirred at 40°C for 12 h, the reaction proceeded to produce amylose, which eluted to the DMSO solution. The time-curse experiment in the system revealed that the enzymatic polymerization took place for 15 min on the inside of the calcium alginate beads and the produced amylose gradually eluted to the surrounding DMSO solution.

One of the significant characteristics in the phosphorylase-catalyzed polymerization is to initiate the reaction from a nonreducing end of the primer [9]. Therefore, the modified primers can be used for the phosphorylase-catalyzed polymerization to introduce the functional groups at the chain end of amylose or maltooligosaccha-

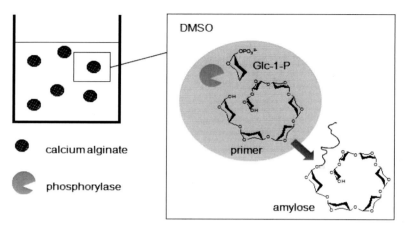

Figure 4.2   Apparent production of enzymatically synthesized amylose in DMSO by means of calcium alginate hydrogel beads/DMSO system.

rides. For example, the phosphorylase-catalyzed polymerization using 2-chloro-4-nitrophenyl (CNP) β-maltopentaoside was performed to produce CNP-maltooligosaccharides with longer chain lengths of DPs in the range 8–11 [10]. These maltooligosaccharide derivatives were indispensable tools in the study on the binding sites and the actions of α-amylases having longer binding area than that of human α-amylase.

Glycogen is known as a high-molecular-weight and water-soluble polysaccharide, which is composed of linear chains containing an average of 10–14 (1→4)-linked α-glucose residues, interlinked by α-(1→6)-glycosidic linkages to form highly branched structure [11,12]. Besides glycogen being a substrate for the *in vivo* phosphorolysis by glycogen phosphorylase, it was used as a primer for the phosphorylase-catalyzed polymerization. When the phosphorylase-catalyzed polymerization of glycogen using Glc-1-P was carried out (Fig. 4.3a), followed by standing further at room temperature for 24 h, the reaction mixture turned into a hydrogel form (Fig. 4.3b) [13]. The hydrogelation was probably caused by the formation of junction zones based on the double helix structure of the elongated amylose chains among the glycogen molecules.

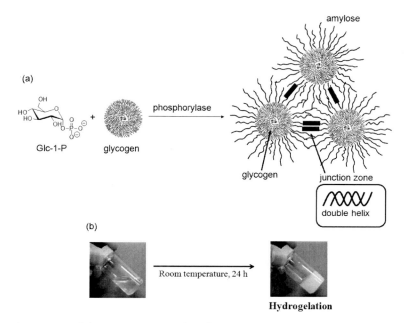

(a)

Glc-1-P   glycogen   phosphorylase   amylose   glycogen   junction zone   double helix

(b)

Room temperature, 24 h

Hydrogelation

Figure 4.3   Schematic reaction for phosphorylase-catalyzed polymerization of glycogen to form hydrogels (a) and photographs of
reaction mixtures before and after hydrogelation (b).

Figure 4.4 shows the stress–strain curves under compression
mode of the glycogen-based hydrogels obtained under the conditions
of various glycogen/Glc-1-P feed ratios: (1)~(5). The condition of (1)
(lower ratio of glycogen to Glc-1-P) gave the elastic gel, but the gels
became stronger and further turned brittle in nature with increasing
the ratios of glycogen to Glc-1-P. The junction zones became
stiffer with increasing the glycogen/Glc-1-P ratio, resulting in the
strengthened gels; however, further increasing the ratio induced the
brittle nature.

The hydrogels were facilely converted into xerogels by
lyophilization of the hydrogels.

The X-ray diffraction (XRD) profile of the xerogel showed
diffraction peaks at 2θ = 15.3, 17.1, 20.0, and 23.0° owing to the
crystalline structure of the double helix amylose chains (Fig. 4.5). This
result indicated that the networks in the xerogel were constructed
based on the double helical entanglement of the elongated amylose

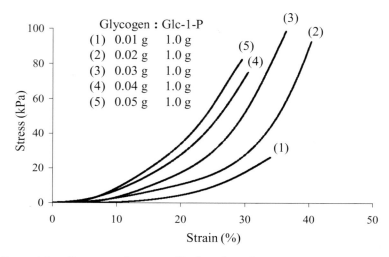

Figure 4.4   Stress–strain curve of hydrogels under compressive mode.

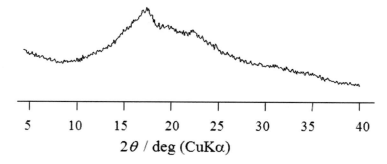

Figure 4.5   XRD profile of xerogel.

chains, which in turn supported the presence of the junction zones by the double helix formation in the hydrogel.

An aqueous solution of the xerogel, which was prepared by dissolution in NaOH aq., followed by neutralization with acetic acid to pH 5.5–6.5 (Fig. 4.6a), gradually turned into the hydrogel form as shown in Fig. 4.6b. These cycles were able to be repeated up to five times. When the standard iodine–iodide solution was added to the neutralized solution immediately after it was prepared by the same procedure as above and the resulting mixture was kept standing, the re-hydrogelation did not take place (Fig. 4.6c). In this

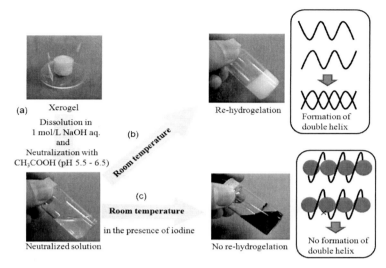

Figure 4.6 Dissolution of xerogel (a), re-hydrogelation (b), and suppression of re-hydrogelation in the presence of iodine (c).

experiment, iodine was included by the elongated amylose chain to form the well-known amylose/iodine inclusion complex, which suppressed the formation of the double helix as the junction zone.

References

1. Kitamura, S. (1996). Starch, polymers, natural and synthetic, In *The Polymeric Materials Encyclopedia, Synthesis, Properties and Applications* (Salamone, C., ed), Vol. 10 (CRC Press, NY), pp. 7915–7922.

2. Gidley, M. J., and Bulpin, P. V. (1989). Aggregation of amylose in aqueous systems: The effect of chain length phase behavior and aggregation kinetics, *Macromolecules,* **22,** pp. 341–346.

3. Niemann, C., Sanger, W., Pfannemüller, B., Eigner, W. D., and Huber, A. (1991). Phospholytic synthesis of low-molecular-weight amyloses with modified terminal groups; comparison of potato phosphorylase and muscle phosphorylase b, In: (Comstock, M. J., ed.), *ACS Symposium Series* (ACS Books Advisory Board), pp. 189–204.

4. Takata, H., Takaha, T., Okada, S., Takagi, M., and Imanaka, T. (1998). Purification and characterization of α-glucan phosphorylase from *Bacillus stearothermophilus, J. Ferment. Bioeng.,* **85**, pp. 156–161.

5. Boeck, B., and Schinzel, R. (1996). Purification and characterization of an α-glucan phosphorylase from the thermophilic bacterium *Thermus thermophilus*, *Eur. J. Biochem.*, **239**, pp. 150–155.

6. Xavier, K. B., Peist, R., Kossmann, M., Boos, W., and Santos, H. (1999). Maltose metabolism in the hyperthermophilic archaeon *Thermococcus litoralis*: Purification and characterization of key enzymes, *J. Bacteriol.*, **181**, pp. 3358–3367.

7. Takaha, T., Yanase, M., Takata, H., and Okada, S. (2001). Structure and properties of *Thermus aquaticus* α-glucan phosphorylase expressed in *Escherichia coli.*, *J. Appl. Glycosci.*, **48**, pp. 71–78.

8. Izawa, H., Kaneko, Y., and Kadokawa, J. (2009). Apparent production of enzymatically synthesized amylose in DMSO by means of calcium alginate hydrogel beads/DMSO system, *J. Carbohydr. Chem.*, **28**, pp. 179–190.

9. Kitamura, S., Yunokawa, H., Mitsuie, S., and Kuge, T. (1982). Study on polysaccharide by the fluorescence method. II. Micro-brownian motion and conformational change of amylose in aqueous solution, *Polym. J.*, **14**, pp. 93–99.

10. Kandra, L., Gyémánt, G., Pál, M., Petró, M., Remenyik, J., and Lipták, A. (2001). Chemoenzymatic synthesis of 2-chloro-4-nitrophenyl β-maltoheptaoside acceptor-products using glycogen phosphorylase b, *Carbohydr. Res.*, **333**, pp. 129–136.

11. Calder, P. C. (1991). Glycogen structure and biogenesis, *Int. J. Biochem.*, **23**, pp. 1335–1352.

12. Manners, D. J. (1991). Recent developments in our understanding of glycogen structure, *Carbohydr. Polym.*, **16**, pp. 37–82.

13. Izawa, H., Nawaji, M., Kaneko, Y., and Kadokawa, J. (2009). Preparation of glycogen-based polysaccharide materials by phosphorylase-catalyzed chain elongation of glycogen, *Macromol. Biosci.*, **9**, pp. 1098–1104.

Chapter 5

Chemoenzymatic Synthesis of Amylose-Grafted Synthetic Polymers by Utilizing Phosphorylase Catalysis

5.1 Outlines of Chemoenzymatic Synthesis of Amylose-Grafted Synthetic Polymers by Utilizing Phosphorylase Catalysis

As the natural polysaccharides such as amylose are recycled carbon resources and considered to be eco-friendly substances [1,2], it is expected that the use of the polysaccharides as one component of hybrid polymers will lead to the production of environmentally benign materials.

Graft copolymer is one of the hybrid polymers widely applied in the industrial fields [3], and has the structure of polymer main chain as a backbone covalently linked to graft chains as branches. However, graft copolymers containing polysaccharides have only been obtained in limited cases. As examples of such materials, a type of graft copolymers composed of polysaccharide main chains and synthetic polymer graft chains is common [4,5]. However, little has been reported regarding preparation of graft copolymers containing polysaccharide graft chains. Because the solubility of polysaccharides is generally poor in any organic solvents, direct

Engineering of Polysaccharide Materials: By Phosphorylase-Catalyzed Enzymatic Chain-Elongation
Jun-ichi Kadokawa and Yoshiro Kaneko
Copyright © 2013 Pan Stanford Publishing Pte. Ltd.
ISBN 978-981-4364-45-4 (Hardcover), ISBN 978-981-4364-46-1 (eBook)
www.panstanford.com

reaction of polysaccharides with polymeric main chains is quite difficult.

Therefore, by means of the combination of the enzymatic polymerization forming amylose, as described in Chapter 4, with a chemical reaction, i.e., a chemoenzymatic approach, several research groups have developed amylose-grafted polymeric materials with well-defined structures (Fig. 5.1) [6,7]. "Macromonomer method" and "polymer reaction method" are generally known as the preparation methods for the amylose-grafted polymers. One of the synthetic routes for the macromonomer methods is that the maltooligosaccharide primer first reacts with the polymerizable compound(monomer) to obtain the maltooligosaccharide-containing monomer (macromonomer) (ii), polymerization of the resulting macromonomer or copolymerization of this macromonomer with

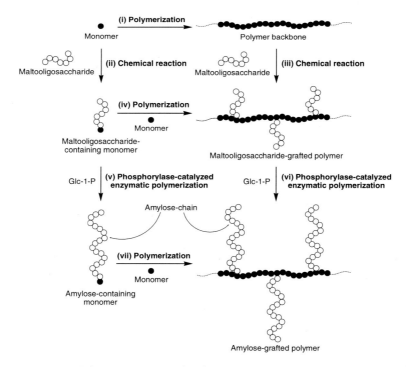

Figure 5.1   Schematic reaction for chemoenzymatic synthesis of amylose-grafted polymers by means of phosphorylase-catalyzed enzymatic polymerization.

comonomer is carried out to produce the maltooligosaccharide-grafted polymer (iv), and then the phosphorylase-catalyzed enzymatic polymerization of Glc-1-P from the resulting graft copolymer is performed to yield the amylose-grafted polymer (vi). As another synthetic route for macromonomer method, after the phosphorylase-catalyzed enzymatic polymerization of Glc-1-P from the maltooligosaccharide-containing monomer, which is obtained by the aforementioned chemical reaction (ii), is conducted to obtain the amylose-containing monomer (macromonomer) (v), (co)polymerization of this macromonomer is performed to produce the amylose-grafted polymer (vii). However, the synthetic route for polymer reaction method is that polymerization of the monomer is first performed (i), the maltooligosaccharide primer reacts with the resulting polymer backbone to obtain the maltooligosaccharide-grafted polymer (iii), and then the phosphorylase-catalyzed enzymatic polymerization of Glc-1-P is carried out as described earlier (vi). In the chemoenzymatic method, the length of amylose graft chain can be controlled by changing the feed ratio of Glc-1-P to the primer on the enzymatic polymerization (v and vi), whereas the number of amylose graft chain can be controlled by changing the feed ratio of the maltooligosaccharide-containing monomer to the comonomer (iv), amylose-containing monomer to the comonomer (vii), and the maltooligosaccharide to the unit number of the polymer main chain (iii).

5.2 General Chemical Reactions to Link Maltooligosaccharide to Polymer Backbones or Polymerizable Groups

Representative three chemical reactions to link the maltooligosaccharides to polymer backbones or polymerizable groups are described in Fig. 5.2.

The reducing end of a maltooligosaccharide can be easily converted to the corresponding aldonic acid by oxidation, which spontaneously leads to an aldonolactone by dryness. The aldonolactone reacts with the amino group to obtain the corresponding aldonamide without protection of hydroxy groups on the maltooligosaccharide (Fig. 5.2a) [8]. Use of amine-functionalized polymer

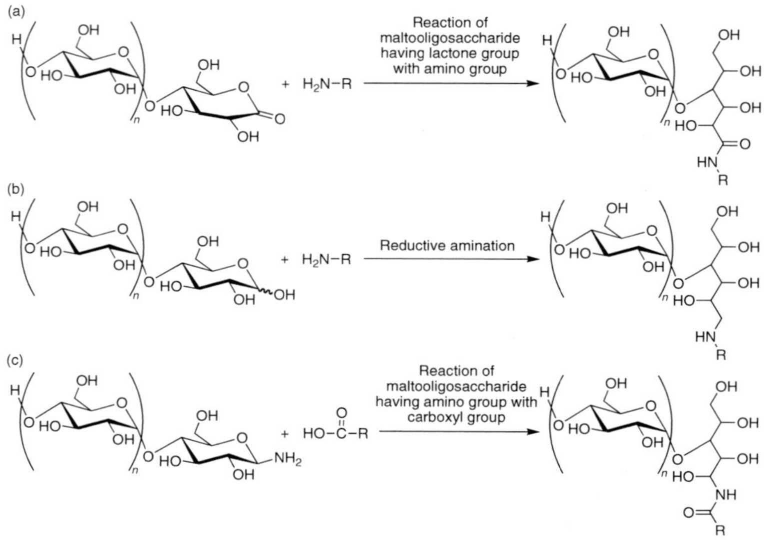

Figure 5.2 Representative chemical reactions to link the maltooligosaccharide to polymer backbones or polymerizable groups.

backbones or polymerizable groups on this reaction can provide maltooligosaccharide-grafted polymer backbones or macromonomers having maltooligosaccharide components.

Reductive amination is a process wherein amine reacts with aldehyde or ketone to form imine, which is subsequently reduced to amine in the presence of reductant (Fig. 5.2b) [9]. Reductive amination can be utilized to link amine-functionalized molecules to maltooligosaccharides because the reducing end of maltooligosaccharide has a hemiacetal structure, which is in equilibrium with an aldehyde group. Sodium cyanoborohydride ($NaBH_3CN$) and sodium triacetoxyborohydride ($NaBH(OCOCH_3)_3$) are generally employed as reductants for the reductive amination of the reducing ends in oligosaccharides under mild conditions.

Introduction of amino group to the reducing end of maltooligosaccharide can be achieved by treatment with aqueous ammonium hydrogen carbonate [10]. The resulting glycosyl amine can be condensed with the carboxyl group via the formation of an amide linkage (Fig. 5.2c).

5.3 Chemoenzymatic Synthesis of Amylose-Grafted Polystyrene

In the research field of the synthetic polymer chemistry, polystyrene and its derivatives are the most representative synthetic polymers because of some unique properties that make them useful in a wide range of products [11]. The commercial success of polystyrene is due to transparency, ease of fabrication, thermal stability, relative high modulus, and low cost. Hybridization between polystyrene and amylose is a promising research topic from the viewpoints of not only preparation of new hybrid materials but also fusion of two symbolic polymers in both synthetic and natural polymer chemistries. However, it may be difficult to hybridize the polystyrene and amylose by blend method of these two polymers because of the immiscibility of these polymeric chains caused by quite different polarities. Therefore, the chemoenzymatic method according to the following reaction manners was investigated to provide such a polystyrene–amylose hybrid material, i.e., an amylose-grafted polystyrene.

The amylose-grafted polystyrene was prepared by two different approaches from a styrene-type macromonomer having a maltooligosaccharide chain, which was obtained by the reaction of a Glc_5 lactone with 4-vinylbenzylamine (Fig. 5.3) [12,13]. In route I, the phosphorylase-catalyzed enzymatic polymerization of Glc-1-P from the macromonomer was first performed to give a styrene-type macromonomer having an amylose chain. The radical polymerization of the product gave the desired amylose-grafted polystyrene. This is indicated as the synthetic route (ii)→(v)→(vii) in Fig. 5.1. In route II, however, the radical polymerization of the macromonomer having a maltooligosaccharide chain was first carried out, followed by the phosphorylase-catalyzed enzymatic polymerization, giving rise to the amylose-grafted polystyrene. This is explained as the synthetic route (ii)→(iv)→(vi) in Fig. 5.1. Every repeating unit in the produced polystyrene derivative by route I has the amylose chains, whereas the amylose chains are probably present partially in the repeating units of the polystyrene derivative obtained by route II because of the probable occurrence of the enzymatic polymerization from a part of the maltooligosaccharide primers on the polystyrene main chain due to steric hindrance in the latter case.

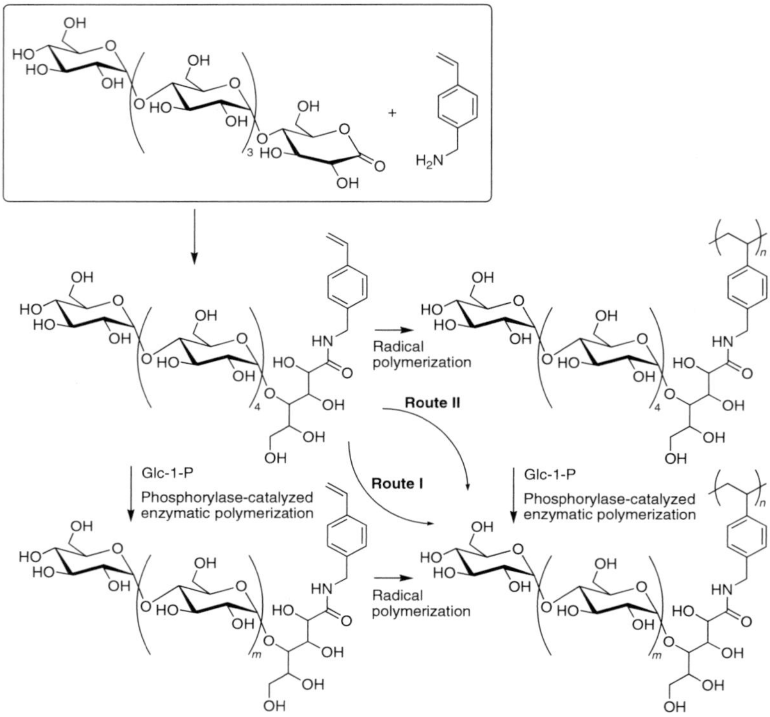

Figure 5.3 Chemoenzymatic synthesis of amylose-grafted polystyrene by means of phosphorylase-catalyzed enzymatic polymerization.

In addition, the phosphorylase-catalyzed enzymatic polymerization was also performed using poly[styrene-*block*-(4-vinylbenzyl maltohexaoside)] as the primer-grafted polystyrene, which was prepared by a two-step 2,2,6,6-tetramethylpiperidine-1-oxyl (TEMPO)–mediated living radical polymerization of styrene and 4-vinylbenzyl maltohexaoside, to afford poly[styrene-*block*-(styrene-*graft*-amylose)] [14].

5.4 Chemoenzymatic Synthesis of Amylose-Grafted Polyacetylene

Researches concerning conjugated polymers have attracted much attention in terms of the various practical applications of their interesting electrical and optical properties [15,16]. Moreover, interests and applications of the conjugated polymers have been extended to the biological fields. In order to endow the conjugated polymers with the biological functions derived from sugar residues, e.g., the sugar-substituted conjugated polymers were synthesized by using the conjugated main chain structures of polyaniline [17], polyisocyanide [18], polythiophene [19], poly(*p*-phenylene) [20,21], poly(*p*-phenylene ethynylene) [22], and poly(*p*-phenylene vinylene) [23]. In the series of these studies, the synthesis of poly(*N*-propargylamide) with galactose residues was investigated [24,25]. It contained a *cis*-polyacetylene main chain and was obtained by the Rh-catalyzed polymerization of a corresponding *N*-propargylamide monomer. On the basis of the aforementioned study, the polyacetylene having graft saccharide chains with higher degree of polymerization (DP), e.g., natural polysaccharides, would be functional polymers with hybrid properties of polyacetylene and polysaccharide. Therefore, the synthesis of the amylose-grafted polyacetylene by the chemoenzymatic method as an effective preparation method for the polyacetylene–polysaccharide hybrid was investigated.

Amylose-grafted polyacetylenes were synthesized by both the macromonomer and polymer reaction methods (Fig. 5.4). In the macromonomer method (Fig. 5.4a) [26], an acetylene-type macromonomer having a maltooligosaccharide chain was polymerized by Rh catalyst to give a polyacetylene with pendant maltooligosaccharide graft chains. Moreover, the Rh-catalyzed copolymerization of the macromonomer with another acetylene monomer was also carried out. However, the DPs of the products obtained by both the aforementioned polymerization and copolymerization were not high (ca. 10), probably owing to the steric hindrance of the bulky oligosaccharide graft chains in the macromonomer and the produced polyacetylene derivatives. The phosphorylase-catalyzed enzymatic polymerization of Glc-1-P from the maltooligosaccharide graft chains on these polyacetylene derivatives was performed to yield two types of the amylose-grafted polyacetylenes (homopolyacetylene and copolyacetylene). These methods are indicated as the synthetic route (ii)→(iv)→(vi) in Fig. 5.1. The complex formation with iodine has been a well-known characteristic property of amylose [27].

Accordingly, the colorless solutions of the amylose-grafted poly-acetylenes in DMSO turned into violet by adding a standard iodine–iodide solution to the polymer solutions, as the same color change in the complex formation of amylose with iodine. The values of the λ_{max} in the UV–vis spectra of the iodine complexes with the amylose graft chains on the homopolyacetylene and copolyacetylene main chains, and a sole amylose, were 577.0, 586.5, and 586.5 nm, respectively; the sole amylose was prepared by the phosphorylase-catalyzed po-lymerization of Glc-1-P using Glc_7 as a primer under the same con-ditions as those for the amylose-grafted polyacetylenes. These data indicated that the average DP of the amylose graft chains on the co-polyacetylene was probably comparable to that of the sole amylose, whereas the average DP of the amylose graft chains on the homopol-yacetylene might be lower in comparison with the sole amylose. On the basis of the aforementioned results, the following difference in the manners during the enzymatic polymerization using the maltoo-ligosaccharide-grafted homopolyacetylene and copolyacetylene was assumed. The enzymatic polymerization was hardly initiated from all the potential sites of the maltooligosaccharide primers on the homopolyacetylene main chain due to steric hindrance, resulting in the lower average DP. However, the less-hindered orientation of the maltooligosaccharide primers on the copolyacetylene main chain was probably more suitable for initiation from most of the potential sites for the enzymatic polymerization.

To obtain the amylose-grafted polyacetylene with higher DP of the main chain, the approach according to the polymer reaction method was conducted (Fig. 5.4b) [28]. First, the reaction of a Glc_7 lactone with an amine-functionalized polyacetylene with high DPs (ca. 72-112) was performed, giving rise to a maltooligosaccharide-grafted polyacetylene. Then, the phosphorylase-catalyzed polymerization from the maltooligosaccharide primers on the polyacetylene derivative was carried out to produce the desired amylose-grafted polyacetylene with high DPs, which was explained as the synthetic route (i)→(iii)→(vi) in Fig. 5.1.

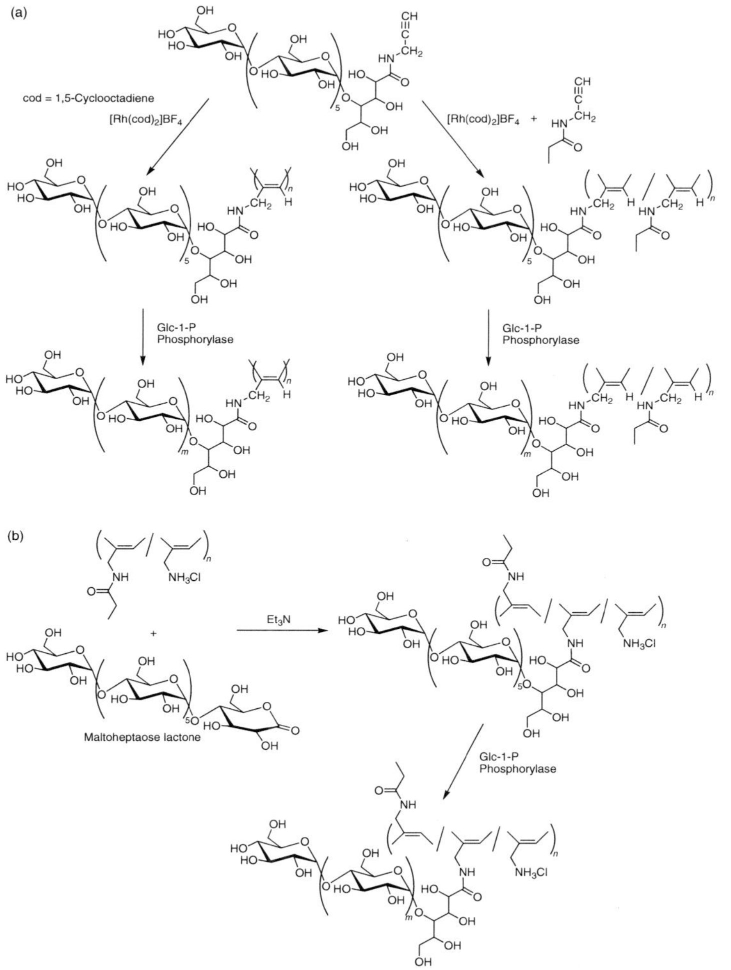

Figure 5.4 Chemoenzymatic synthesis of amylose-grafted polyacetylenes by means of phosphorylase-catalyzed enzymatic polymerization by macromonomer method (a) and polymer reaction method (b).

5.5 Chemoenzymatic Synthesis of Amylose-Grafted Poly(Vinyl Alcohol)

Poly(vinyl alcohol) (PVA) film exhibits unique properties such as formation of a complex with iodine, which has attracted much attention in terms of application as a polarizing material for liquid crystal displays (LCDs). The polarized film in LCD is generally prepared based on the PVA/iodine complex [29,30]. However, because iodine is easily released from the PVA backbone under relatively high temperature and/or high humidity conditions, this film is susceptible to heat and moisture. Therefore, the PVA-based polarized film is practically used by being sandwiched between protecting films such as triacetylcellulose (TAC) films. Development of a sole film, which has an ability to stably retain iodine without the use of the protecting film, is hopefully expected.

Amylose is a well-known host compound that forms a stable inclusion complex with iodine [31]. Therefore, a blend film composed of PVA and amylose is possibly one of the candidates for such a new polarized film stably retaining iodine without the use of TAC [32,33]. However, the blend film may have heterogeneous distribution of amylose chains in PVA matrix due to their aggregation. To obtain such a film stably retaining iodine, a PVA derivative covalently bonded to amylose, e.g., an amylose-grafted PVA, was prepared.

An amylose-grafted PVA was synthesized by the chemoenzymatic method (Fig. 5.5) [34]. First, Glc$_7$ was introduced to an amine-functionalized PVA by the reductive amination using NaBH$_3$CN

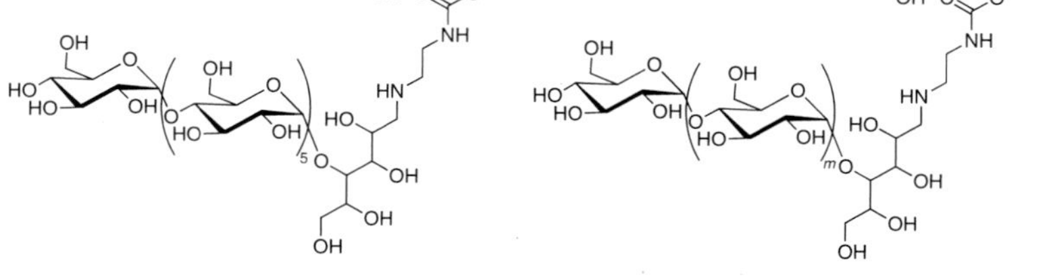

Figure 5.5 Chemoenzymatic synthesis of amylose-grafted poly(vinyl alcohol) by means of phosphorylase-catalyzed enzymatic polymerization.

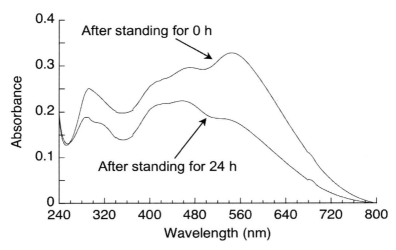

Figure 5.6 UV–vis spectra of the iodine-doped films of amylose-grafted PVA.

to produce a maltooligosaccharide-grafted PVA. Then, the phosphorylase-catalyzed enzymatic polymerization of Glc-1-P from the maltooligosaccharide graft chains on the PVA main chain was conducted to obtain the amylose-grafted PVA. This synthetic route is explained as (i)→(iii)→(vi) in Fig. 5.1. A film of the product was soaked in an iodine–iodide ethanol solution to form an iodine-doped film. The UV–vis analysis of the doped film indicated that iodine was retained in this film even after it was left standing for 24 h (Fig. 5.6). This was probably because the iodide ions were contained in the cavities of the amylose graft chains in this film.

5.6 Chemoenzymatic Synthesis of Amylose-Grafted Polydimethylsiloxane

The chemoenzymatic approach by utilizing the phosphorylase-catalyzed enzymatic polymerization was applied to the preparation of amylose-grafted inorganic polymeric materials such as polydimethylsiloxanes (PDMSs) [35]. PDMSs have various interesting properties, e.g., high oxygen permeability, low toxicity, and biocompatibility, which are advantages as practical biomaterials

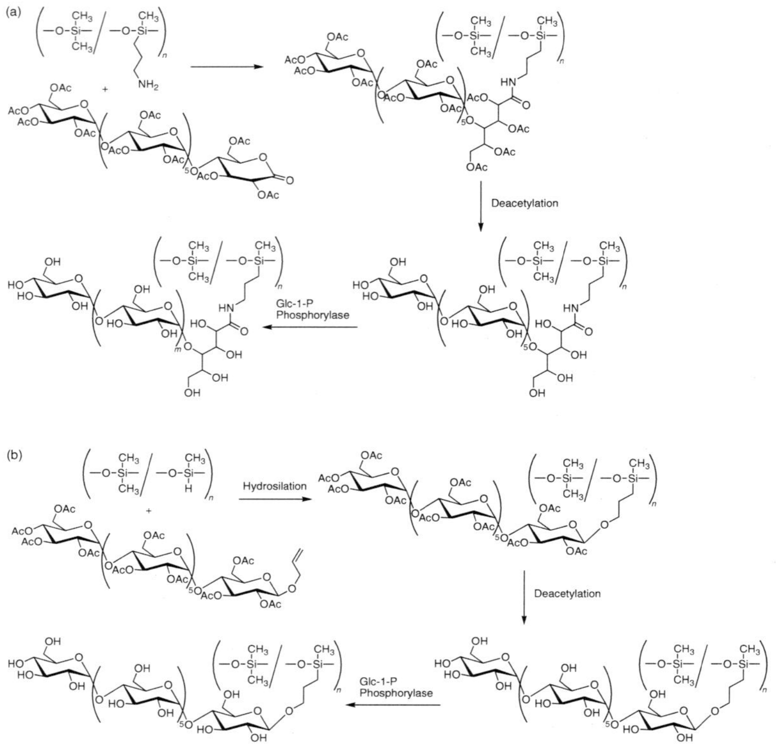

Figure 5.7 Chemoenzymatic synthesis of amylose-grafted polydimethylsiloxanes using Glc$_7$ lactone derivative (a) and allylated Glc$_7$ (b) by means of phosphorylase-catalyzed enzymatic polymerization.

[36]. Therefore, saccharide–PDMS hybrids would be expected to have a significant potential for biological applications.

Therefore, amylose-grafted PDMSs were synthesized as follows [37,38]. First, maltooligosaccharide-grafted PDMSs were prepared by the reaction of a Glc$_7$ lactone derivative with an amine-functionalized PDMS (Fig. 5.7a) or the hydrosilylation of an allylated Glc$_7$ with a PDMS derivative having Si–H linkage (Fig. 5.7b), followed by deacetylation. Then, the phosphorylase-catalyzed polymerization of Glc-1-P using the maltooligosaccharide-grafted PDMSs was carried out to give the amylose-grafted PDMSs. These are indicated as the synthetic route (i)→(iii)→(vi) in Fig. 5.1.

5.7 Chemoenzymatic Synthesis of Amylose-Grafted Silica Gel

The chiral recognition ability of amylose derivatives is one of the significant functions for their practical use of the amylose-conjugated materials [39]. On the basis of this viewpoint, silica gel bounded by amylose through the phosphorylase-catalyzed enzymatic polymerization was prepared, and the chiral recognition ability of its phenylcarbamate derivative was investigated [40].

Two kinds of synthetic approaches are illustrated in Figs. 5.8 and 5.9. In approach (I), Glc$_5$ lactone was first prepared, followed by reaction with 3-aminopropyltriethoxysilane to obtain the maltooligosaccharide bearing triethoxysilyl group. Amylose chains were then extended by the phosphorylase-catalyzed enzymatic polymerization, and the resulting amylose derivative was allowed to react with silica gel to produce amylose-grafted silica gel (Fig. 5.8). In approach (II), Glc$_5$ was first oxidized to be converted into a potassium gluconate at a reducing terminal residue, and the enzymatic polymerization was then performed. After the lactonization, the amylose was immobilized onto the silica gel to obtain amylose-grafted one (Fig. 5.9). Finally, both the amylose-grafted silica gels were treated with a large excess of 3,5-dimethylphenyl isocyanate to derivatize the remaining hydroxy groups of amylose to the carbamates (Figs. 5.8 and 5.9).

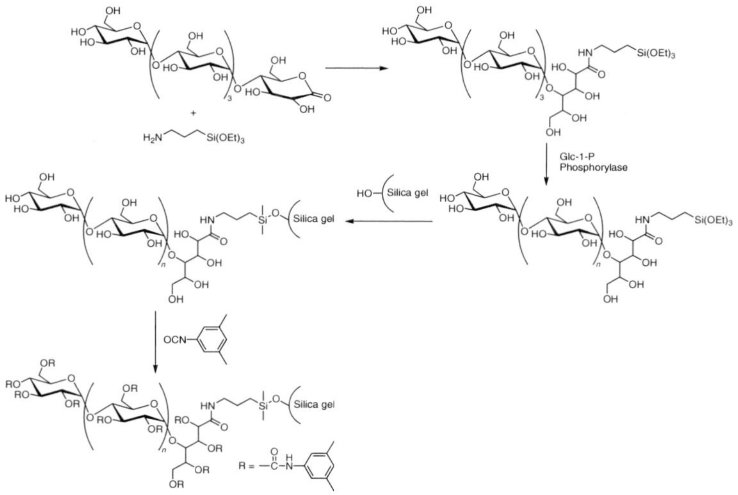

Figure 5.8   Synthetic approach (I) for amylose-grafted silica gel.

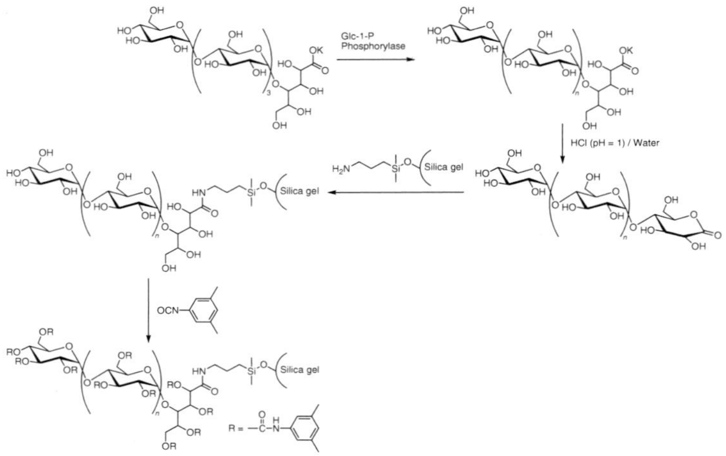

Figure 5.9   Synthetic approach (II) for amylose-grafted silica gel.

The chiral recognition abilities of these materials were investigated using racemic molecules, e.g., *trans*-stilbene oxide by HPLC. Consequently, the enantiomers eluted at different retention times, indicating that racemic *trans*-stilbene oxides were completely separated.

References

1. Rouilly, A., and Rigal, L. (2002). Agro-materials: A bibliographic review, *J. Macromol. Sci. Polym. Rev.*, **C42**, pp. 441–479.

2. Mohanty, A. K., Misra, M., and Drzal, L. T. (2002). Sustainable bio-composites from renewable resources: Opportunities and challenges in the green materials world, *J. Polym. Environ.*, **10**, pp. 19–26.

3. Jenkins, D. W., and Hudson, S. M. (2001). Review of vinyl graft copolymerization featuring resent advances toward controlled radical-based reactions and illustrated with chitin/chitosan trunk polymers, *Chem. Rev.*, **101**, pp. 3245–3273.

4. Wu, Y. D., Liu, C. B., Zhao, X. Y., and Xiang, J. N. (2008). A new biodegradable polymer: PEGylated chitosan-g-PEI possessing a hydroxyl group at the PEG end, *J. Polym. Res.*, **15**, pp. 181–185.

5. Gurruchaga, M., Echeverria, I., and Gonni, I. (2008). Synthesis and rheological characterization of graft copolymers of butyl and hydroxyethyl methacrylates on starches, *J. Appl. Polym. Sci.*, **108**, pp. 4029–4037.

6. Kaneko, Y., and Kadokawa, J. (2009). In *Handbook of Carbohydrate Polymers* (Ito, R., and Matsuo, Y., eds), Nova Science Publishers, Inc., Hauppauge, NY, Chapter 23, pp. 671–691.

7. Kadokawa, J. (2011). Precision polysaccharide synthesis catalyzed by enzymes, *Chem. Rev.*, **111**, 4308–4345.

8. Kobayashi, K., Sumitomo, H., and Itoigawa, T. (1987). Maltopentaose- and maltoheptaose-carrying styrene macromers and their homopolymers, *Macromolecules*, **20**, pp. 906–908.

9. Yalpani, M., and Hall, L. D. (1984). Some chemical and analytical aspects of polysaccharide modifications. 3. Formation of branched-chain, soluble chitosan derivatives, *Macromolecules*, **17**, pp. 272–281.

10. Lubineau, A., Auge, J., and Drouillat, B. (1995). Improved synthesis of glycosylamines and a straightforward preparation of *n*-acylglycosylamines as carbohydrate-based detergents, *Carbohydr. Res.*, **266**, pp. 211–219.

11. Kroschwitz, J. I. (1990). *Concise Encyclopedia of Polymer Science and Engineering*, Wiley Interscience, NY.

12. Kobayashi, K. (1995). Biological functions of synthetic polysaccharides, *Macromol. Symp.*, **99**, pp. 157–167.

13. Kobayashi, K., Kamiya, S., and Enomoto, N. (1996). Amylose-carrying styrene macromonomer and its homo- and copolymers: Synthesis via enzyme-catalyzed polymerization and complex formation with iodine, *Macromolecules*, **29**, pp. 8670–8676.

14. Narumi, A., Kawasaki, K., Kaga, H., Satoh, T., Sugimoto, N., and Kakuchi, T. (2003). Glycoconjugated polymer 6. Synthesis of poly[styrene-block-(styrene-*graft*-amylose)] via potato phosphorylase-catalyzed polymerization, *Polym. Bull.*, **49**, pp. 405–410.

15. Yamamoto, T., and Hayashida, N. (1998). π-Conjugated polymers bearing electronic and optical functionalities. Preparation, properties and their applications, *React. Funct. Polym.*, **37**, pp. 1–17.

16. Stenger-Smith, J. D. (1998). Intrinsically electrically conducting polymers. Synthesis, characterization, and their applications, *Prog. Polym. Sci.*, **23**, pp. 57–79.

17. Kadokawa, J., Shinmen, Y., and Shoda, S. (2005). Synthesis of glucose-containing polyaniline by the oxidative polymerization of *N*-glucosylaniline, *Macromol. Rapid Commun.*, **26**, pp. 103–106.

18. Hasegawa, T., Kondoh, S., Matsuura, K., and Kobayashi, K. (1999). Rigid helical poly(glycosyl phenyl isocyanide)s: Synthesis, conformational

analysis, and recognition by lectins, *Macromolecules*, **32**, pp. 6595–6603.

19. Baek, M. G., Stevens, R. C., and Charych, D. H. (2000). Design and synthesis of novel glycopolythiophene assemblies for colorimetric detection of influenza virus and *E. coli*, *Bioconjugate Chem.*, **11**, pp. 777–788.

20. Yamashita, Y., Kaneko, Y., and Kadokawa, J. (2007). Synthesis of poly(*p*-phenylene)s having alternating sugar and alkyl substituents by Suzuki coupling polymerization and evaluation of their main-chain conformations, *Eur. Polym. J.*, **43**, pp. 3795–3806.

21. Yamashita, Y., Kaneko, Y., and Kadokawa, J. (2007). Synthesis of glucose-substituted poly(*p*-phenylene)s with twisted main-chain in one direction due to induced axial chirality, *Polym. Bull.*, **58**, pp. 635–643.

22. Kim, I. B., Erdogan, B., Wilson, J. N., and Bunz, U. H. F. (2004). Sugar-poly(*p*-phenylene ethynylene) conjugates as sensory materials: Efficient quenching by Hg^{2+} and Pb^{2+} ions, *Chem. Eur. J.*, **10**, pp. 6247–6254.

23. Takasu, A., Iso, K., Dohmae, T., and Hirabayashi, T. (2006). Synthesis of sugar-substituted poly(phenylenevinylene)s, *Biomacromolecules*, **7**, pp. 411–414.

24. Suenaga, M., Kaneko, Y., Kadokawa, J., Nishikawa, T., Mori, H., and Tabata, M. (2006). Amphiphilic poly(*N*-propargylamide) with galactose and lauryloyl groups: Synthesis and properties, *Macromol. Biosci.*, **6**, pp. 1009–1018.

25. Kadokawa, J., Tawa, K., Suenaga, M., Kaneko, Y., and Tabata, M. (2006). Polymerization and copolymerization of a new *N*-propargylamide monomer having a pendant galactose residue to produce sugar-carrying poly(*N*-propargylamide)s, *J. Macromol. Sci. Part A Pure Appl. Chem.*, **43**, pp. 1179–1187.

26. Kadokawa, J., Nakamura, Y., Sasaki, Y., Kaneko, Y., and Nishikawa, T. (2008). Chemoenzymatic synthesis of amylose-grafted polyacetylenes, *Polym. Bull.*, **60**, pp. 57–68.

27. Knutson, C. A. (2000). Evaluation of variations in amylose–iodine absorbance spectra, *Carbohydr. Polym.*, **42**, pp. 65–72.

28. Sasaki, Y., Kaneko, Y., and Kadokawa, J. (2009). Chemoenzymatic synthesis of amylose-grafted polyacetylene by polymer reaction manner and its conversion into organogel with DMSO by cross-linking, *Polym. Bull.*, **62**, pp. 291–303.

29. Yosomiya, T., Suzuki Y., and Yosomiya, R. (1995). Polarization characteristics of poly(vinyl alcohol) films containing metal iodide, *Angew. Makromol. Chem.*, **230**, pp. 171–178.

30. Yang, H., and Horii, F. (2008). Investigation of the structure of poly(vinyl alcohol)–iodine complex hydrogels prepared from the concentrated polymer solutions, *Polymer*, **49**, pp. 785–791.

31. Yu, X. C., Houtman, C., and Atalla, R. H. (1996). The complex of amylose and iodine, *Carbohydr. Res.*, **292**, pp. 129–141.

32. Yang, S. Y., and Huang, C. Y. (2008). Plasma treatment for enhancing mechanical and thermal properties of biodegradable PVA/starch blends, *J. Appl. Polym. Sci.*, **109**, pp. 2452–2459.

33. Wang, J., Lu, Y., Yuan, H. L., and Dou, P. (2008). Crystallization, orientation morphology, and mechanical properties of biaxially oriented starch/polyvinyl alcohol films, *J. Appl. Polym. Sci.*, **110**, pp. 523–530.

34. Kaneko, Y., Matsuda, S., and Kadokawa, J. (2010). Chemoenzymatic synthesis of amylose-grafted poly(vinyl alcohol), *Polym. Chem.*, **1**, pp. 193–197.

35. Kaneko, Y. (2009). In *Interfacial Researches in Fundamental and Material Sciences of Oligo- and Polysaccharides* (Kadokawa, J., ed), Transworld Research Network, Trivandrum, India, Chapter 6, pp. 109–124.

36. Belanger, M. C., and Marois, Y. (2001). Hemocompatibility, biocompatibility, inflammatory and *in vivo* studies of primary reference materials low-density polyethylene and polydimethylsiloxane: A review, *J. Biomed. Mater. Res.*, **58**, pp. 467–477.

37. von Braunmühl, V., Jonas, G., and Stadler, R. (1995). Enzymatic grafting of amylose from poly(dimethylsiloxanes), *Macromolecules*, **28**, pp.17–24.

38. von Braunmühl, V., and Stadler, R. (1996). Polydimethylsiloxanes with amylose side chains by enzymatic polymerization, *Macromol. Symp.*, **103**, pp. 141–148.

39. Okamoto, Y., and Kaida, Y. (1994). Resolution by high-performance liquid-chromatography using polysaccharide carbamates and benzoates as chiral stationary phases, *J. Chromatogr. A.*, **666**, pp. 403–419.

40. Enomoto, N., Furukawa, S., Ogasawara, Y., Akano, H., Kawamura, Y., Yashima, E., and Okamoto, Y. (1996). Preparation of silica gel-bonded amylose through enzyme-catalyzed polymerization and chiral recognition ability of its phenylcarbamate derivative in HPLC, *Anal. Chem.*, **68**, pp. 2798–2804.

Chapter 6

Chemoenzymatic Synthesis of Amylose-Grafted Biopolymers by Utilizing Phosphorylase Catalysis

6.1 Outlines of Chemoenzymatic Synthesis of Amylose-Grafted Biopolymers by Utilizing Phosphorylase Catalysis

Heteropolysaccharides and saccharide–polypeptide conjugates having branched structures are often found in nature. For example, arabinoxylan, gum arabic, and guaran as former [1] and glycoproteins and proteoglycans as latter [2–4] play important roles in living systems. These materials are composed of two or more different kinds of components, which contribute to their prominent functions. On the basis of these viewpoints, the development of an efficient method for the preparation of branched (grafted) artificial heteropolysaccharides and saccharide–polypeptide conjugates is a promising topic in biomaterials research fields. Therefore, the chemoenzymatic synthesis of amylose-grafted biopolymers such as polysaccharides and polypeptide was investigated.

Amylose-grafted biopolymers have been synthesized by the chemoenzymatic method, i.e., the combined method of the phosphorylase-catalyzed enzymatic polymerization with the chemical reaction, as described in Chapter 5 [5–7]. This chemoenzymatic method was achieved by the introduction of maltooligosaccharide primers

Engineering of Polysaccharide Materials: By Phosphorylase-Catalyzed Enzymatic Chain-Elongation
Jun-ichi Kadokawa and Yoshiro Kaneko

to the abundant polysaccharide and polypeptide chains and the subsequent phosphorylase-catalyzed enzymatic polymerization of Glc-1-P (Fig. 5.1).

6.2 Chemoenzymatic Synthesis of Amylose-Grafted Chitin and Chitosan

Chitin, a $(1\rightarrow4)$-linked 2-acetamido-2-deoxy-β-D-glucan, and chitosan, a $(1\rightarrow4)$-linked 2-amino-2-deoxy-β-D-glucan, are the most abundant polysaccharides found in nature [8]. These polysaccharides are regarded to be biodegradable and noncytotoxic, and have some interesting biological activities. However, wide application of these polysaccharides is limited because of their specific properties caused by the regular saccharide chain structures. Therefore, to develop the novel functional heteropolysaccharides based on chitin and chitosan, the preparation of the amylose-grafted polysaccharides was investigated.

Amylose-grafted chitin and chitosan were synthesized by the chemoenzymatic method as follows (Fig. 6.1) [9,10]. First, the Glc$_7$

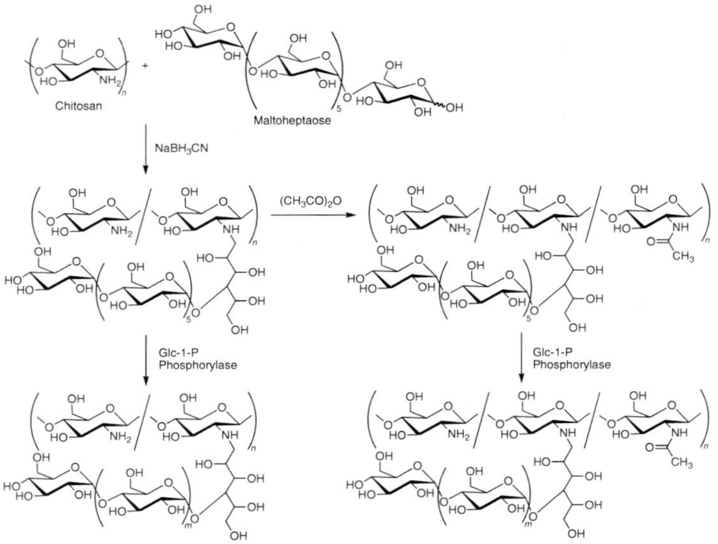

Figure 6.1 Chemoenzymatic synthesis of amylose-grafted chitin and chitosan by means of phosphorylase-catalyzed enzymatic polymerization.

primer was introduced to chitosan by the reductive amination using NaBH$_3$CN in a mixed solvent of aqueous acetic acid/methanol to give a maltooligosaccharide-grafted chitosan. This material was converted into a maltooligosaccharide-grafted chitin by *N*-acetylation using acetic anhydride. Then, the phosphorylase-catalyzed enzymatic polymerization of Glc-1-P from the maltooligosaccharide primers on these chitin and chitosan derivatives was performed to obtain the amylose-grafted chitin and chitosan.

The amylose-grafted chitin and chitosan were insoluble in any solvents, e.g., aqueous acetic acid and DMSO, which were good solvents for chitosan and amylose, respectively. The XRD patterns of these materials showed typical *A*-type crystalline structures owing to amyloses (Fig. 6.2). Such crystalline structures are generally

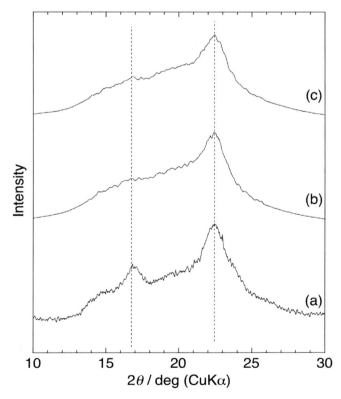

Figure 6.2   XRD patterns of amylose (a), amylose-grafted chitosan (b), and amylose-grafted chitin (c).

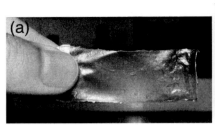
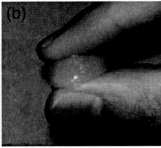

Figure 6.3   Photographs of a film (a) and a hydrogel (b) obtained from amylose-grafted chitosan.

attributed to the formation of a double helix of amylose [11]. Therefore, it is assumed that one of the reasons for the insolubility of these materials is probably caused by molecular aggregation as a result of this crystalline structure. The aggregation in the material would contribute its conversion into film and hydrogel forms (Fig. 6.3). For example, the hydrogel of the amylose-grafted chitosan could be formed by drying the reaction mixture slowly in the vessel at 40–50°C.

6.3   Chemoenzymatic Synthesis of Amylose-Grafted Cellulose

Two representative natural polysaccharides, cellulose and amylose, are composed of the same structural unit, i.e., the glucose unit, but linked through the different $(1{\rightarrow}4)$-β- and $(1{\rightarrow}4)$-α-glucosidic linkages, respectively. The roles of cellulose and amylose in nature are completely different; the former is the structural material and the latter acts as the energy source. In this section, the chemoenzymatic synthesis of the graft heteropolysaccharide composed of these two polysaccharides, i.e., amylose-grafted cellulose, is described [12]. This material has a very interesting and unique structure because it is composed of two polysaccharide chains with the same structural unit but with different linkages.

For the preparation of the desired amylose-grafted cellulose by the chemoenzymatic method as shown in Fig. 6.4, the amino groups have necessarily been introduced to cellulose by the reductive

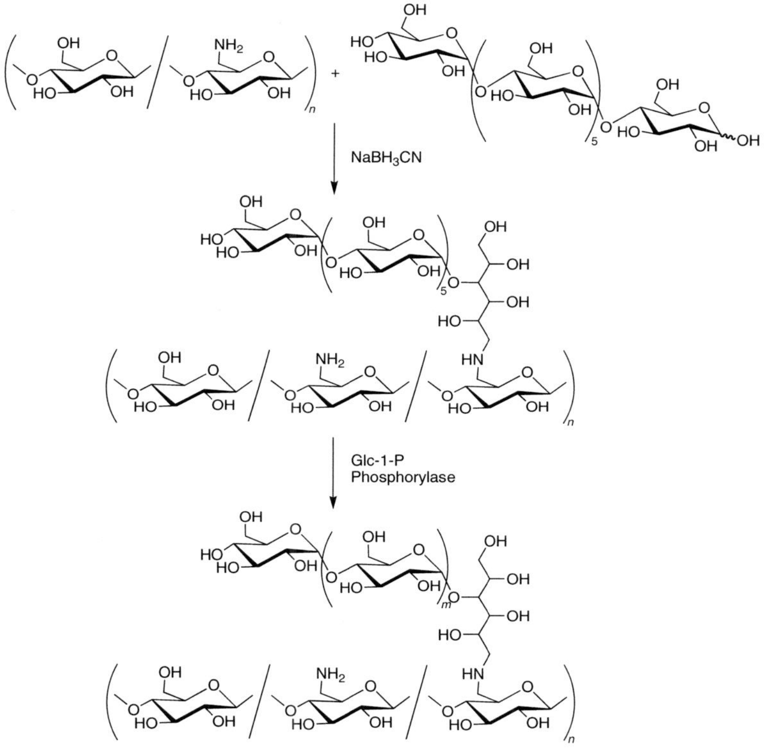

Figure 6.4 Chemoenzymatic synthesis of amylose-grafted cellulose by means of phosphorylase-catalyzed enzymatic polymerization.

amination, giving rise to the maltooligosaccharide-grafted cellulose. Therefore, the synthesis of amine-functionalized cellulose was first performed, which was successfully obtained by three reaction steps, i.e., the partial tosylation of the OH groups at C-6 positions, the displacement of the tosylates by the azido groups, and the reduction to the amino groups (Fig. 6.5).

The reductive amination of the amine-functionalized cellulose with maltoheptaose was carried out by a reaction procedure same as that of chitosan with maltoheptaose as aforementioned. Subsequently, the synthesis of the amylose-grafted cellulose was performed by the phosphorylase-catalyzed enzymatic polymerization of Glc-1-P from the maltooligosaccharide graft chains on cellulose (Fig. 6.4).

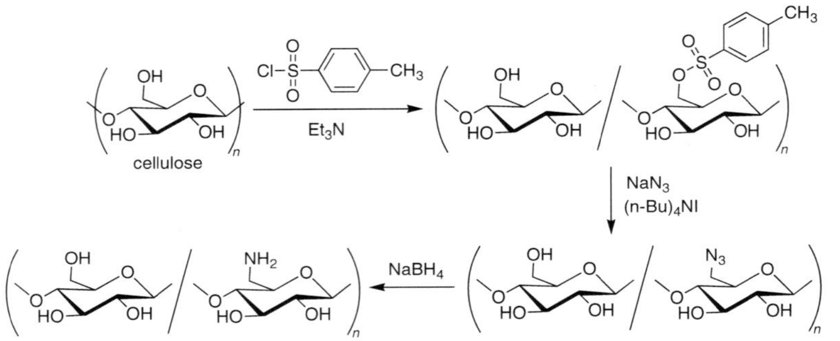

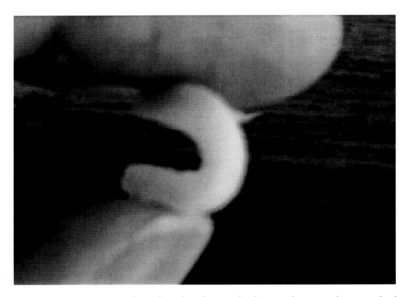

Figure 6.5   Synthesis of amine-functionalized cellulose.

When the reaction mixture obtained by the enzymatic polymerization was kept in a Petri dish at room temperature for around five days, it totally turned into gel form (Fig. 6.6). The produced gel was washed with water several times to remove some contaminants such as the unreacted Glc-1-P. This gel has a more tough nature than that formed from the amylose-grafted chitosan as described earlier.

Figure 6.6   Photograph of gel obtained from the amylose-grafted cellulose.

6.4   Chemoenzymatic Synthesis of Amylose-Grafted Anionic Polysaccharides

The water-soluble anionic polysaccharides such as alginic acid and xanthan gum are representative hydrocolloids, which are used as a stabilizer, a viscous agent, and a structure provider in food industries. To develop the functional hydrocolloids, the chemoenzymatic method was extended to alginic acid as an anionic polysaccharide [13] to give the amylose-grafted alginate (Fig. 6.7) [14]. Alginic acid is a linear polysaccharide composed of (1→4)-linked β-D-mannuronate and (1→4)-linked α-L-guluronate units. For this approach, an amine-functionalized maltooligosaccharide was chemically introduced into sodium alginate by condensation with carboxylates of the alginate to produce a maltooligosaccharide-grafted alginate. Then, the phosphorylase-catalyzed enzymatic polymerization of Glc-1-P from the maltooligosaccharide primers on the alginate main chain was conducted to produce the amylose-grafted alginate.

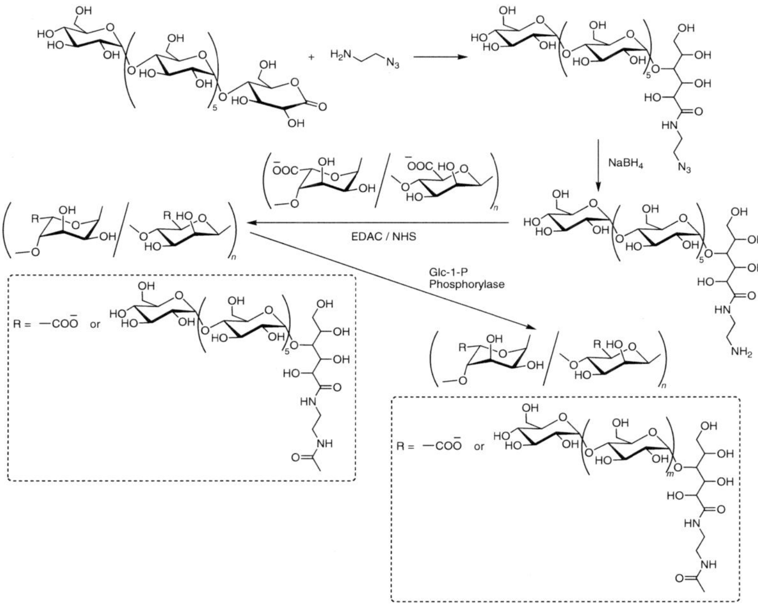

Figure 6.7   Chemoenzymatic synthesis of amylose-grafted alginate by means of phosphorylase-catalyzed enzymatic polymerization.

The preparation of beads from the resulting amylose-grafted alginate was attempted by adding its alkaline solution into calcium chloride aqueous solution. Consequently, beads were obtained from the amylose-grafted alginate containing shorter amylose graft chains (DP < 50), whereas that containing longer amylose graft chains (DP = 100) did not afford the formation of beads. This result indicated that the longer amylose graft chains attached to the alginate main-chain disturbed the formation of the stable matrices composed of the cross-linked calcium alginates, resulting in difficulty in the formation of beads. In addition, enzymatic disintegradability of the beads was investigated by β-amylase-catalyzed reaction. When the beads obtained from the amylose-grafted alginate containing shorter amylose graft chains were kept standing in the presence of β-amylase in a stirred acetate buffer at 40°C for 6 h, the solution gradually became turbid, indicating disintegration of the beads.

The chemoenzymatic method was also investigated using another anionic polysaccharide, i.e., xanthen gum, as a main-chain of amylose-grafted polymer. Xanthan gum, which is a water-soluble polysaccharide produced by *Xanthomonas campestris*, is a representative food hydrocolloid [15]. It has a cellulose-type main-chain (β-(1→4)-glucan) with trisaccharide side-chains (mannose-β-(1→4)-glucuronic acid-β-(1→2)-mannose-α-(1→3)-) attached to alternate glucose units in the main-chain [16]. The α-mannoside unit is acetylated at position 6 and the β-mannoside unit is partially pyruvated at positions 4 and 6. Because the side-chain contains carboxylate groups, xanthan gum is an anionic polysaccharide.

The chemoenzymatic synthesis of an amylose-grafted xanthan gum was performed as follows (Fig. 6.8) [17]. An amine-function-alized maltooligosaccharide was chemically introduced to xanthan gum by condensation with its carboxylates using a condensing agent to produce a maltooligosaccharide-grafted xanthan gum. Then, a phosphorylase-catalyzed enzymatic polymerization of Glc-1-P from the graft chain ends on the xanthan gum derivative was performed, giving an amylose-grafted xanthan gum.

The product formed a gel with an ionic liquid, which was converted into a hydrogel with high water content by replacement of the ionic liquid with water. The ionically cross-linked hydrogel was also provided by soaking the primary formed hydrogel in $FeCl_3$ aqueous solution. When the mechanical properties of the ionically cross-linked hydrogels with Fe^{3+} were evaluated by compressive

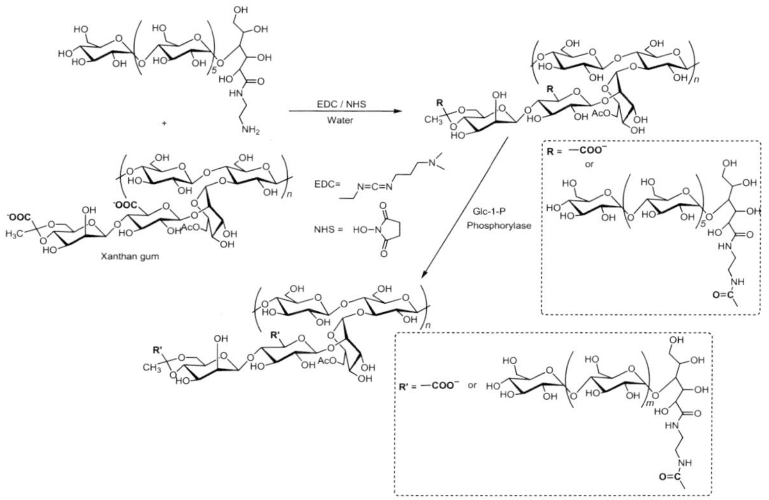

Figure 6.8   Chemoenzymatic synthesis of amylose-grafted xanthan gum by means of phosphorylase-catalyzed enzymatic polymerization.

testing, the fracture strain values increased with increasing the functionalities or DPs of the amylose graft chains, whereas the fracture stress values were mostly unchanged regardless of the functionalities or DPs. It can be considered that the Fe^{3+}-treated hydrogels of the amylose-grafted xanthan gums are constructed by not only the ionically cross-linking with Fe^{3+} and the double-helix conformation of xanthan gum chains but also the double helix conformation of amylose graft chains, because amylose is also known to readily form the double-helix conformation. The presence of the double-helix structure between amylose graft chains probably contributed to the formation of looser network structure in the hydrogels, resulting in the enhancement of the fracture stress values.

6.5   Chemoenzymatic Synthesis of Amylose-Grafted Polypeptide

Glycoproteins, peptidoglycans, and proteoglycans are saccharide–polypeptide conjugates, which occur in blood, plasma membranes, intercellular matrixes, and connective tissues. These naturally occurring saccharide–polypeptide conjugates play important roles in various kinds of biological processes [4]. Oligosaccharide–polypeptide conjugates have been prepared by many researchers to develop model compounds for molecular recognition [18]. On the basis of these researches, as a new model compound for biological applications, the preparation of polysaccharide–polypeptide conjugate, i.e., amylose-grafted poly(L-glutamic acid), by chemoenzymatic method was investigated (Fig. 6.9) [19].

First, maltopentaosylamine was condensed with the pendant carboxyl groups of poly(L-glutamic acid) using a condensing agent to give a maltopentaose-grafted poly(L-glutamic acid). Then, the phosphorylase-catalyzed polymerization of Glc-1-P from the maltooligosaccharide primers on the poly(L-glutamic acid) main-chain was performed to produce the amylose-grafted poly(L-glutamic acid). The maltopentaose-grafted poly(L-glutamic acid) formed a helical conformation at lower pH and a random coil conformation at higher pH. However, little α-helix content was observed for the amylose-grafted poly(L-glutamic acid), indicating that the helical formation was disturbed by the amylose chains, probably owing to steric hindrance.

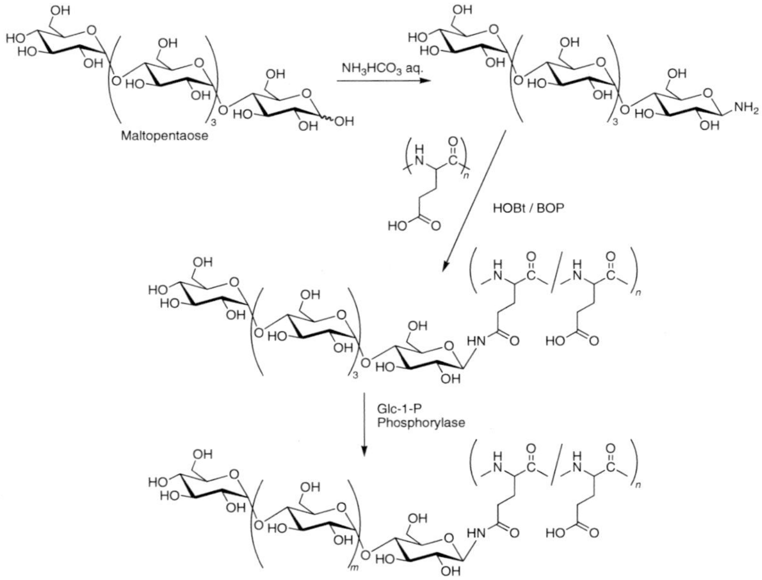

Figure 6.9 Chemoenzymatic synthesis of amylose-grafted poly(L-glutamic acid) by means of phosphorylase-catalyzed enzymatic polymerization.

References

1. Shuerch, C. (1986). Polysaccharides, In *Encyclopedia of Polymer Science and Engineering*, 2nd ed., John Wiley & Sons, NY, pp. 87–162.

2. Bernfield, M., Götte, M., Park, W. P., Reizes, O., Fitzgerald, M. L., Lincecum, J., and Zako, M. (1999). Functions of cell surface heparan sulfate proteoglycans, *Annu. Rev. Biochem.*, **68**, pp. 729–777.

3. Iozzo, R. V. (2005). Basement membrane proteoglycans: From cellar to ceiling, *Nat. Rev. Mol. Cell Biol.*, **6**, pp. 646–656.

4. Montreuil, J., Vliegenthart, J. F. G., and Schachter, H. (1995). *New Comprehensive Biochemistry* (Neuberger, A., and van Deenen, L. L. M., eds), Vol. 29, Elsevier, Amsterdam, Netherlands.

5. Kaneko, Y., and Kadokawa, J. (2008). Biomacromolecules as organic resources, *J. Soc. Rubber Ind. Jpn.*, **81**, pp. 112–117.

6. Kaneko, Y., and Kadokawa, J. (2009). In *Handbook of Carbohydrate Polymers* (Ito, R., and Matsuo, Y., eds), Nova Science Publishers, Inc., Hauppauge, NY, Chapter 23, pp. 671–691.

7. Kadokawa, J. (2011). Precision polysaccharide synthesis catalyzed by enzymes, *Chem. Rev.*, **111**, 4308–4345.

8. Rathke, T. D., and Hudson, S. M. (1994). Review of chitin and chitosan as fiber and film formers, *J. Macromol. Sci. Rev. Macromol. Chem. Phys.*, **C34**, pp. 375–437.

9. Matsuda, S., Kaneko, Y., and Kadokawa, J. (2007). Chemoenzymatic synthesis of amylose-grafted chitosan, *Macromol. Rapid Commun.*, **28**, pp. 863–867.

10. Kaneko, Y., Matsuda, S., and Kadokawa, J. (2007). Chemoenzymatic syntheses of amylose-grafted chitin and chitosan, *Biomacromolecules*, **8**, pp. 3959–3964.

11. Zobel, H. F. (1988). Starch crystal transformations and their industrial importance, *Starch/Stärke*, **40**, pp. 1–7.

12. Omagari, Y., Matsuda, S., Kaneko, Y., and Kadokawa, J. (2009). Chemoenzymatic synthesis of amylose-grafted cellulose, *Macromol. Biosci.*, **9**, pp. 450–455.

13. Prasad, K., and Kadokawa, J. (2009). In *Alginates: Biology and Applications* (Rehm, B. H. A., ed), Springer, Berlin, pp. 175–210.

14. Omagari, Y., Kaneko, Y., and Kadokawa, J. (2010). Chemoenzymatic synthesis of amylose-grafted alginate and its formation of enzymatic disintegratable beads, *Carbohydr. Polym.*, **82**, pp. 394–400.

15. Jansson, P. E., Kenne, L., and Lindberg, B. (1975). Structure of the extracellular polysaccharide from xanthomonas campestris, *Carbohydr. Res.*, **45**, pp. 275–282.

16. Melton, L. D., Mindt, L., and Rees, D. A. (1976). Covalent structure of the extracellular polysaccharide from *Xanthomonas campestris*: Evidence from partial hydrolysis studies, *Carbohydr. Res.*, **46**, pp. 245–257.

17. Arimura, T., Omagari, Y., Yamamoto, K., and Kadokawa, J. (2011). Chemoenzymatic synthesis and hydrogelation of amylose-grafted xanthan gums, *Int. J. Biol. Macromol.*, **49**, 498–503.

18. Kobayashi, K., Tawada, E., Akaike, T., and Usui, T. (1997). Artificial glycopolypeptide conjugates: Simple synthesis of lactose- and *N,N'*-diacetylchitobiose-substituted poly(L-glutamic acid)s through N-β-glycoside linkages and their interaction with lectins, *Biochim. Biophys. Acta-Gen. Subj.*, **1336**, pp. 117–122.

19. Kamiya, S., and Kobayashi, K. (1998). Synthesis and helix formation of saccharide-poly(L-glutamic acid) conjugates, *Macromol. Chem. Phys.*, **199**, pp. 1589–1596.

Chapter 7

Preparation of Amylose–Polymer Inclusion Complexes in Phosphorylase-Catalyzed Enzymatic Polymerization ("Vine-Twining Polymerization")

7.1 Outlines of Vine-Twining Polymerization

Amylose is a well-known host molecule that readily forms inclusion complexes with slender guest molecules having relatively lower molecular weight by hydrophobic interaction between guest molecules and the cavity of amylose [1–7]. However, little had been reported regarding the formation of inclusion complexes composed of amylose and polymeric compounds [8–14]. The principal difficulty for incorporating polymeric materials into the cavity of amylose is that the driving force for the binding is only due to weak hydrophobic interactions. Amylose, therefore, does not have the sufficient ability to include the long chains of polymeric guests into its cavity.

By means of the phosphorylase-catalyzed enzymatic polymerization of Glc-1-P for direct construction of amylose as described in the earlier chapters, the method for the preparation of inclusion complexes composed of amylose and synthetic polymers has been developed. The representation of this reaction system is similar to the way that vines of plants grow twining around a rod. Accordingly, it has been proposed that this polymerization method for

Engineering of Polysaccharide Materials: By Phosphorylase-Catalyzed Enzymatic Chain-Elongation
Jun-ichi Kadokawa and Yoshiro Kaneko
Copyright © 2013 Pan Stanford Publishing Pte. Ltd.
ISBN 978-981-4364-45-4 (Hardcover), ISBN 978-981-4364-46-1 (eBook)
www.panstanford.com

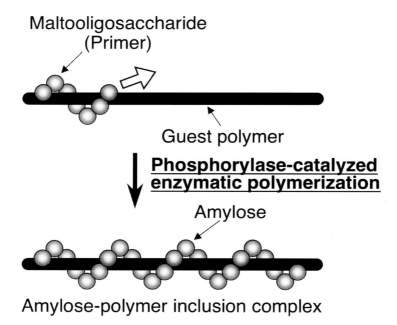

Figure 7.1   Image of "vine-twining polymerization."

the preparation of amylose–polymer inclusion complexes is named "vine-twining polymerization" (Fig. 7.1) [15–24]. In this chapter, the procedure, the principal result, and the proposed mechanism for the vine-twining polymerization are described.

7.2   Preparation of Amylose–Poly(Tetrahydrofuran) Inclusion Complex

First example of the method leading to an amylose–polymer inclusion complex was achieved by amylose-forming polymerization in the presence of poly(tetrahydrofuran) (PTHF) (M_n = 4000) as a guest polymer [25]. The phosphorylase-catalyzed enzymatic polymerization of Glc-1-P from Glc_7 as the primer was performed in the presence of a telechelic PTHF with hydroxy end groups in sodium citrate buffer at ca. 40°C (Fig. 7.2a). The resulting product was isolated and characterized by means of XRD and ^1H NMR measurements. The XRD pattern of the product (Fig. 7.3a) was completely different from that of amylose (Fig. 7.3b) and PTHF, and was similar to that of the inclusion complexes of amylose with monomeric compounds, as shown in an earlier study [26].

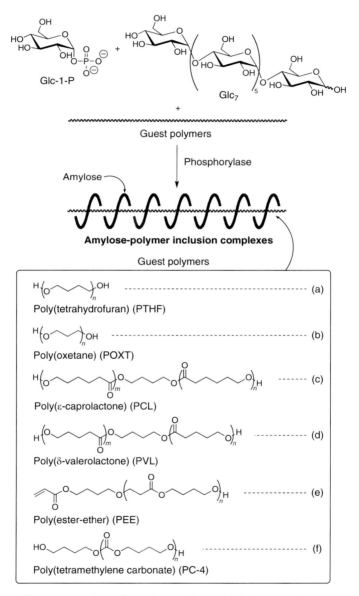

Figure 7.2 Preparation of amylose–polymer inclusion complexes by vine-twining polymerization.

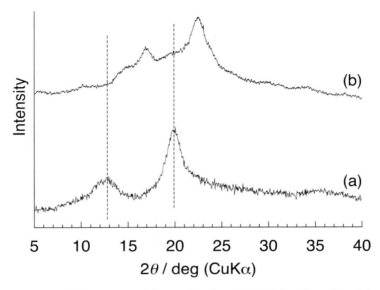

Figure 7.3   XRD patterns of the product from PTHF (a) and amylose (b).

The ^{1}H NMR spectrum in DMSO-d_6 of the product showed signals owing to not only amylose but also PTHF (Fig. 7.4), in spite of washing with methanol, which is a good solvent of PTHF. Furthermore, the methylene peak of PTHF was broadened and shifted upfield compared to that of the original PTHF. This is because each methylene group of PTHF is immobile and interacts with the protons inside the amylose cavity. When PTHF was added to the NMR sample of the product in DMSO-d_6, two different signals due to methylene protons of PTHF were observed. This result suggested that the PTHF of the product was in an environment different from an original PTHF unit. To further confirm the structure of the product, spin-lattice relaxation time (T_1) measurements were investigated, as T_1 measurements of inclusion complexes have often been used for the identification of their structures. In general, the T_1 values of the inclusion complexes are shorter than those of the corresponding individual molecules. Actually, the T_1 value of the methylene peak of the PTHF in the product was shorter than that of the original PTHF. The shorter T_1 in the product indicated restriction of the methylene movement due to the included conditions.

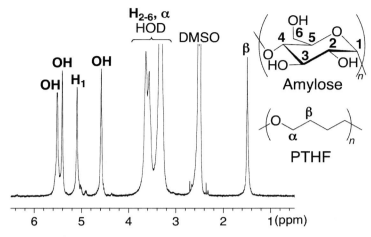

Figure 7.4 ^{1}H NMR spectrum in DMSO-d_6 of the product from PTHF.

In addition, a similar NMR pattern was also observed in NaOD/D$_2$O solvent (Fig. 7.5). The original PTHF was insoluble in NaOD/D$_2$O, and no peak owing to PTHF appeared in the ^{1}H NMR spectrum of the suspension of PTHF in NaOD/D$_2$O. The PTHF in the product was probably solubilized in the alkaline solution by its inclusion in the cavity of amylose. These XRD and NMR data supported the conclusion that the helical inclusion complexes were synthesized.

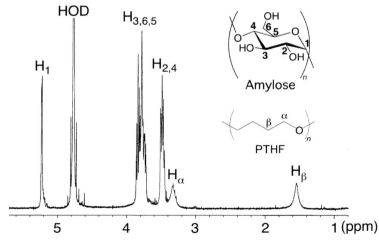

Figure 7.5 ^{1}H NMR spectrum in NaOD/D$_2$O (1.0 mol/L) of the product from PTHF.

Generally, one helical turn of amylose is composed of approximately six repeating glucose units when linear molecules of small cross-sectional area, e.g., fatty acids, are included [27]. The repeat distance of the helix of amylose was reported as ca. 0.80 nm [27], whereas the length of one unit of PTHF was calculated as ca. 0.60 nm (see Fig. 7.6). Therefore, 4.5 repeating glucose units in amylose correspond to the length of one PTHF unit (Fig. 7.6). On the basis of these calculations, the ratio of the proton numbers between amylose and PTHF in the ideal inclusion complex can be calculated. The integrated ratio of the signal due to amylose to the signal due to PTHF in the ^{1}H NMR spectrum of the product was in good agreement with the calculated value [25]. This also supported the structure of the inclusion complex.

The molecular weights of the amylose and PTHF in the inclusion complex were evaluated by means of ^{1}H NMR measurements when

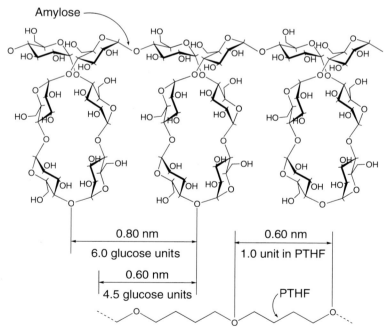

Figure 7.6   Illustration of repeat distance of amylose helix and unit length of PTHF.

the molecular weight of PTHF equal to 4000 was used. The molecular weight of the amylose was 12200–14600, corresponding to 9.9–11.9 nm of molecular length in helical form. However, the molecular weight of the included PTHF was ca. 2800, suggesting that the chain length is ca. 23.0 nm. Therefore, one PTHF molecule is probably included by two amylose molecules on the average.

Mixing amylose and PTHF in a buffer did not form the inclusion complex. This observation suggested that the inclusion complex formed during enzymatic polymerization. To study the relation between the formation of the inclusion complex and the enzymatic polymerization process, the following experiment was performed (Fig. 7.7). When PTHF was added to the reaction solution immediately after the general enzymatic polymerization of Glc-1-P had started, an identical inclusion complex to that mentioned earlier was obtained. However, the contents of PTHF in the products decreased as the time between the start of the enzymatic polymerization and the addition of the PTHF to the solution was increased. These observations revealed that the inclusion complexes were not formed after the production of amyloses with relatively higher molecular weights. These results indicated that polymerization proceeded with the formation of the inclusion complex.

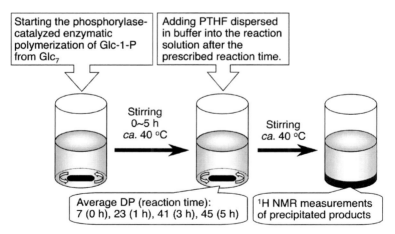

Figure 7.7 Investigation of relation between the formation of the inclusion complex and phosphorylase-catalyzed enzymatic polymerization process.

Preparation of inclusion complexes using PTHFs with various M_ns (1000, 2000, 10,000, and 14,000) was also performed [28]. When PTHFs with M_ns = 1000 and 2000 were used as the guest polymers, inclusion complexes were obtained, which were confirmed by means of the XRD and ^{1}H NMR measurements. In contrast, PTHFs with higher M_ns, such as 10,000 and 14,000, were not dispersed well in the buffer of the polymerization solvent, and accordingly, inclusion complexes were not formed from these PTHFs. To obtain the inclusion complexes using these PTHFs, the polymerization was performed in the following two-phase system. The PTHF was dissolved in diethyl ether and the buffer was added to the solution (1:5, v/v). Enzymatic polymerization of Glc-1-P then occurred with vigorous stirring to disperse the diethyl ether phase in the buffer. The XRD patterns of the products from the PTHFs with M_ns equal to 10,000 and 14,000 obtained by the two-phase system indicated the formation of the inclusion complexes.

The effect of the end groups of the telechelic PTHFs as the guest polymers was investigated [28]. The end groups employed were the hydroxy (–OH, as aforementioned), methoxy (–OCH$_3$), ethoxy (–OCH$_2$CH$_3$), and benzyloxy (–OCH$_2$Ph) groups. The content of PTHF in the product obtained from the methoxy-terminated PTHF was close to that obtained from the hydroxy-terminated PTHF, indicating the formation of the inclusion complex. However, the content of PTHF in the product obtained from the ethoxy-terminated PTHF was much lower than that obtained from the aforementioned guest PTHFs. In addition, when the benzyloxy-terminated PTHF was used, no inclusion complex was obtained. These results indicated that the formation of the inclusion complexes was strongly affected by the bulkiness of the end groups of the PTHFs.

7.3 Preparation of Inclusion Complex Using Other Polyethers as Guest Polymers

To investigate the effect of the alkyl chain lengths of the guest polyethers for the formation of inclusion complexes, the enzymatic polymerization was carried out in the presence of polyethers with different alkyl chain lengths, i.e., PTHF (Fig. 7.2a), poly(oxetane) (POXT, Fig. 7.2b), and poly(ethylene glycol) (PEG) [28]. The structures of the products were characterized by means of the XRD and ^{1}H NMR measurements. The XRD profiles of the product from POXT showed the same pattern as that from PTHF. Furthermore, the ^{1}H NMR spectrum of the product in DMSO-d_6 showed the signals due to both amylose and POXT. These observations indicated that the inclusion complex was formed by using POXT as the guest polyether. However, the XRD pattern of the product obtained with PEG was similar to that of amylose. In addition, the peak due to PEG was not observed in the ^{1}H NMR spectrum of the product. No formation of the inclusion complex with PEG was detected from these analytical data. This was probably attributed to the hydrophilicity of PEG, which caused less hydrophobic interaction between PEG and the cavity of amylose. These results indicated that the hydrophobicity of the guest polymers was an important factor for the formation of the inclusion complexes in this type of polymerization system.

7.4 Preparation of Amylose–Polyester Inclusion Complexes

Since the importance of the hydrophobicity of the guest polymers was found, hydrophobic polyesters as guest polymers such as telechelic poly(ε-caprolactone)s (PCLs) and telechelic poly(δ-valerolactone)s (PVLs) were employed for the preparation of amylose–polyester inclusion complexes [29,30]. The phosphorylase-catalyzed enzymatic polymerization of Glc-1-P from Glc$_7$ was performed in the presence of the polyesters in the sodium citrate buffer (Fig. 7.2c,d). The resulting products were characterized by means of ^{1}H NMR and XRD measurements, which supported the structures of the inclusion complexes. When PCL with higher molecular weight (M_n = 2000) was used as the guest polymer for the experiment same as the aforementioned, the PCL was not dispersed well in the citrate buffer, and accordingly, the inclusion complex was not formed. To be dispersed in the reaction solvent, the polymerization was conducted in a mixed solvent of citrate buffer with acetone (5:1, v/v). The obtained product was characterized by means of the ^{1}H NMR and XRD measurements to be the inclusion complex. The inclusion complex was formed in citrate buffer by using PVL with a molecular weight of 2000, indicating that the PVLs had more advantageous properties as guest polymers for the formation of the inclusion complexes in the citrate buffer compared with the PCLs.

The IR spectrum of the PVL in the product (Fig. 7.8a) was compared with that of the original PVL (Fig. 7.8b), and showed that no crystalline PVL existed in the product, owing to the inclusion of the PVL chain into the cavity of amylose. This was in good agreement with the XRD data, in which the XRD profile of PVL showed strong crystalline peaks, whereas no such peaks were observed at all in the XRD profile of the product. The same results were obtained in the IR and XRD analyses of the product from PCL.

As the other guest polyester, a hydrophobic poly(ester-ether) (PEE) was employed in the formation of the inclusion complex [30]. The preparation of the inclusion complex using PEE was attempted in an experimental manner similar to that using the above polyesters (Fig. 7.2e). The structure of the product was determined by means of the ^{1}H NMR and XRD measurements to be the inclusion complex. When the hydrophilic poly(ester-ether) ($-CH_2CH_2C(=O)OCH_2CH_2O-$) was used as the guest polymer, no inclusion complex was formed. This result indicated that the hydrophobicity of the guest polymers strongly affected the formation of the inclusion complexes.

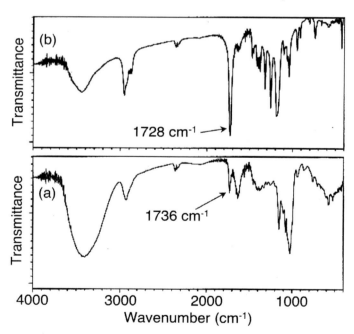

Figure 7.8 IR spectra of the product obtained from PVL (a) and the original PVL (b).

7.5 Preparation of Amylose–Polycarbonate Inclusion Complexes

The aforementioned guest polymers contain the relative polar linkages in the main-chains and do not have the side groups. Taking this into consideration, aliphatic polycarbonates as guest polymers for the vine-twining polymerization were employed, giving rise to the corresponding inclusion complexes with amylose [31]. The four hydrophobic polycarbonates with different methylene chain lengths were used, which were poly(tetramethylene carbonate) (PC-4), poly(octamethylene carbonate) (PC-8), poly(decamethylene carbonate) (PC-10), and poly(dodecamethylene carbonate) (PC-12).

First, PC-4 was investigated as a guest polycarbonate for the vine-twining polymerization. The preparation of an amylose–PC-4 inclusion complex was carried out under the conditions almost same as those using polyethers and polyesters as guest polymers described earlier (Fig. 7.2f). The precipitated product was characterized by means of the ^{1}H NMR, XRD, and IR measurements, which supported the structures of amylose–PC-4 inclusion complex. In addition, the structure of the product was investigated by means of the differential scanning calorimetry (DSC) measurement. In the DSC thermogram of PC-4, an endothermic peak corresponding to the melting (T_m) was observed (Fig. 7.9a), whereas any thermal transition is not observed in the DSC trace of the product (Fig. 7.9b). These DSC traces supported that no crystalline PC-4 existed in the product.

The effect of the methylene chain lengths in the polycarbonates was investigated on the formation of the inclusion complexes in this polymerization system using PC-4, PC-8, PC-10, and PC-12 as the guest molecules. One helical turn of amylose is composed of about six repeating glucose units and the repeat distance of the helix of amylose has been reported as ca. 0.80 nm as aforementioned, whereas the lengths of one unit of PC-4, PC-8, PC-10, and PC-12 were calculated to be ca. 0.84, 1.38, 1.65, and 1.92 nm, respectively (Fig. 7.10). On the basis of the aforementioned calculations, the ratios of the proton numbers between H-1 of amylose to β or γ of PC-4, PC-8, PC-10, and PC-12 ([β or γ]/H-1) in the inclusion complexes were

(b)
(a)
Endotherm
T_m of PC-4
40
50
60
70
80
90
100
Temperature (°C)

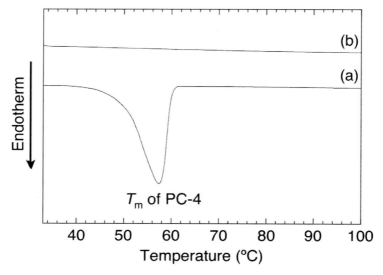

Figure 7.9 DSC traces of PC-4 (a) and the product obtained from PC-4 (b).

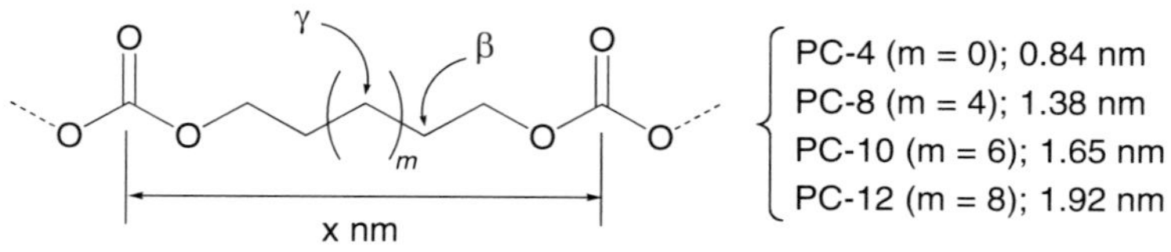

γ
β
O
O
O
O
O
O
m
x nm
PC-4 (m = 0); 0.84 nm
PC-8 (m = 4); 1.38 nm
PC-10 (m = 6); 1.65 nm
PC-12 (m = 8); 1.92 nm

Figure 7.10 Lengths of one unit of polycarbonates.

found to be 0.63, 0.77, 0.97, and 1.11, respectively. The integrated ratio of these two signals in the ^{1}H NMR spectrum of the product obtained using PC-4 was 0.65, which was in good agreement with the calculated value. However, that of the product obtained using PC-8 (0.55) was slightly smaller than the calculated value. However, the values of the products obtained using PC-10 and PC-12 were 0.23 and 0.20, respectively, which were obviously lower than the calculated values. The guest polycarbonates having longer methylene chain lengths were probably aggregated in the aqueous buffer/acetone mixed solvent, and accordingly, separated from the cavity of amylose, causing the difficulty of complex formation.

References

1. Kim, O. K., Choi, L. S., Zhang, H. Y., He, X. H., and Shih, Y. H. (1996). Second-harmonic generation by spontaneous self-poling of supramolecular thin films of an amylose–dye inclusion complex, *J. Am. Chem. Soc.*, **118**, pp. 12220–12221.

2. Choi, L. S., and Kim, O. K. (1998). Unusual thermochromic behavior of photoreactive dyes confined in helical amylose as inclusion complex, *Macromolecules*, **31**, 9406–9408.

3. Lalush, I., Bar, H., Zakaria, I., Eichler, S., and Shimoni, E. (2005). Utilization of amylose–lipid complexes as molecular nanocapsules for conjugated linoleic acid, *Biomacromolecules*, **6**, pp. 121–130.

4. Sanji, T., Kato, N., Kato, M., and Tanaka, M. (2005). Helical folding in a helical channel: Chiroptical transcription of helical information through chiral wrapping, *Angew. Chem.-Int. Ed.*, **44**, pp. 7301–7304.

5. Sanji, T., Kato, N., and Tanaka, M. (2006). Chirality control in oligothiophene through chiral wrapping, *Org. Lett.*, **8**, pp. 235–238.

6. Kim, O. K., Je, J., and Melinger, J. S. (2006). One-dimensional energy/electron transfer through a helical channel, *J. Am. Chem. Soc.*, **128**, pp. 4532–4533.

7. Sanji, T., Kato, N., and Tanaka, M. (2006). Switching of optical activity in oligosilane through pH-responsive chiral wrapping with amylose, *Macromolecules*, **39**, p. 75087512.

8. Shogren, R. L., Greene, R. V., and Wu, Y. V. (1991). Complexes of starch polysaccharides and poly(ethylene-*co*-acrylic acid) – Structure and stability in solution, *J. Appl. Polym. Sci.*, **42**, pp. 1701–1709.

9. Shogren, R. L. (1993). Complexes of starch with telechelic poly(ε-caprolactone) phosphate, *Carbohydr. Polym.*, **22**, pp. 93–98.

10. Ikeda, M., Furusho, Y., Okoshi, K., Tanahara, S., Maeda, K., Nishino, S., Mori, T., and Yashima, E. (2006). A luminescent poly(phenylenevinylene)-amylose composite with supramolecular liquid crystallinity, *Angew. Chem.-Int. Ed.*, **45**, pp. 6491–6495.

11. Kida, T., Minabe, T., Okabe, S., and Akashi, M. (2007). Partially-methylated amyloses as effective hosts for inclusion complex formation with polymeric guests, *Chem. Commun.*, pp. 1559–1561.

12. Kida, T., Minabe, T., Nakano, S., and Akashi, M. (2008). Fabrication of novel multilayered thin films based on inclusion complex formation between amylose derivatives and guest polymers, *Langmuir*, **24**, pp. 9227–9229.

13. Frampton, M. J., Claridge, T. D. W., Latini, G., Brovelli, S., Cacialli, F., and Anderson, L. (2008). Amylose-wrapped luminescent conjugated polymers, *Chem. Commun.*, pp. 2797–2799.

14. Kaneko, Y., Kyutoku, T., Shimomura, N., and Kadokawa, J. (2011). Formation of amylose–poly(tetrahydrofuran) inclusion complexes in ionic liquid media, *Chem. Lett.*, **40**, pp. 31–33.

15. Kadokawa, J., and Shoda, S. (2003). New methods for Architectures of glyco-materials, *J. Synthetic Org. Chem. Jpn.*, **61**, pp. 1207–1217.

16. Kadokawa, J., and Shoda, S. (2003). Enzymatic synthesis of glyco-macromonomers, *Sen'i Gakkaishi*, **59**, pp. 74–78.

17. Kadokawa, J. (2004). Vine-twining polymerization, *High Polym. Jpn.*, **53**, pp. 591–594.

18. Kaneko, Y., and Kadokawa, J. (2005). Vine-twining polymerization: A new preparation method for well-defined supramolecules composed of amylose and synthetic polymers, *Chem. Rec.*, **5**, pp. 36–46.

19. Kaneko, Y., and Kadokawa, J. (2006). Synthesis of nanostructured bio-related materials by hybridization of synthetic polymers with polysaccharides or saccharide residues, *J. Biomater. Sci. Polym. Edn.*, **17**, pp. 1269–1284.

20. Kaneko, Y., and Kadokawa, J. (2009). In *Modern Trends in Macromolecular Chemistry* (Lee, J. N., ed), Nova Science Publishers, Inc., Hauppauge, NY, Chapter 8, pp. 199–217.

21. Kadokawa, J., and Kobayashi, S. (2010). Polymer synthesis by enzymatic catalysis, *Curr. Opin. Chem. Biol.*, **14**, pp. 145–153.

22. Kaneko, Y., and Kadokawa, J. (2010). Construction of supramolecules based on polysaccharides, *High Polym. Jpn.*, **59**, pp. 405–408.

23. Kaneko, Y., and Kadokawa, J. (2010). Preparation method for polysaccharide supramolecules using amylose-forming polymerization field: Vine-twining polymerization, *Kobunshi Ronbunshu*, **67**, pp. 553–559.

24. Kadokawa, J. (2011). Precision polysaccharide synthesis catalyzed by enzymes, *Chem. Rev.*, **111**, 4308–4345.

25. Kadokawa, J., Kaneko, Y., Tagaya, H., and Chiba, K. (2001). Synthesis of an amylose–polymer inclusion complex by enzymatic polymerization of glucose 1-phosphate catalyzed by phosphorylase enzyme in the presence of polyTHF: A new method for synthesis of polymer-polymer inclusion complexes, *Chem. Commun.*, pp. 449–450.

26. Seneviratne, H. D., and Biliaderis, C. G. (1991). Action of α-amylases on amylose–lipid complex superstructures, *J. Cereal Sci.*, **13**, pp. 129–143.

27. Zobel, H. F. (1988). Starch crystal transformations and their industrial importance, *Starch*, **40**, pp. 1–7.

28. Kadokawa, J., Kaneko, Y., Nagase, S., Takahashi, T., and Tagaya, H. (2002). Vine-twining polymerization: Amylose twines around polyethers to form amylose–polyether inclusion complexes, *Chem. Eur. J.*, **8**, pp. 3321–3326.

29. Kadokawa, J., Kaneko, Y., Nakaya, A., and Tagaya, H. (2001). Formation of an amylose–polyester inclusion complex by means of phosphorylase-catalyzed enzymatic polymerization of α-D-glucose 1-phosphate monomer in the presence of poly(ε-caprolactone), *Macromolecules*, **34**, pp. 6536–6538.

30. Kadokawa, J., Nakaya, A., Kaneko, Y., and Tagaya, H. (2003). Preparation of inclusion complexes between amylose and ester-containing polymers by means of vine-twining polymerization, *Macromol. Chem. Phys.*, **204**, pp. 1451–1457.

31. Kaneko, Y., Beppu, K., and Kadokawa, J. (2008). Preparation of amylose/polycarbonate inclusion complexes by means of vine-twining polymerization, *Macromol. Chem. Phys.*, **209**, pp. 1037–1042.

Chapter 8

Extension of Vine-Twining Polymerization by Phosphorylase Catalysis

8.1 Selective Inclusion of Amylose in Vine-Twining Polymerization

8.1.1 Amylose Selectively Includes One from Mixtures of Two Resemblant Guest Polymers

As described in Chapter 7, hydrophobic polyethers, polyesters, a poly(ester-ether), and polycarbonates having appropriate methylene chain lengths were employed as the guest polymers for the vine-twining polymerization to form the corresponding inclusion complexes with amylose. On the basis of the results in the studies using these guest polymers, the suitable hydrophobicity of the guest polymers had been considered to be a very important factor in whether amylose was include them or not. The aforementioned property of amylose that included limited guest polymers with appropriate hydrophobicity in the vine-twining polymerization was applied to perform the selective inclusion toward two resemblant guest polymers.

For example, the vine-twining polymerization was performed in the presence of a mixture of POXT (M_n = ~1800) and PTHF (M_n

Engineering of Polysaccharide Materials: By Phosphorylase-Catalyzed Enzymatic Chain-Elongation
Jun-ichi Kadokawa and Yoshiro Kaneko
Copyright © 2013 Pan Stanford Publishing Pte. Ltd.
ISBN 978-981-4364-45-4 (Hardcover), ISBN 978-981-4364-46-1 (eBook)
www.panstanford.com

= ~1600) in sodium acetate buffer for 6 h at 40–45°C (Fig. 8.1a) [1,2]. The ^{1}H NMR spectrum of the employed mixture of the guest polyethers (CDCl$_3$) showed that the unit ratio of POXT/PTHF in feed was assessed to be 0.90:1.00 (Fig. 8.2a). However, in the ^{1}H NMR spectrum of the product obtained by the vine-twining polymerization (DMSO-d_6), the signals due to PTHF and amylose were prominently observed and the signal due to POXT slightly appeared (POXT/PTHF = 0.02:1.00) (Fig. 8.2b). When POXT or PTHF was independently used as the guest for the vine-twining polymerization, the inclusion complex was formed well as described in Chapter 7 [3]. These results indicated that amylose almost selectively included PTHF from a mixture of the two resemblant polyethers in the vine-twining polymerization. The slight difference in the hydrophobicities of two polyethers probably caused the difference in the inclusion by amylose toward them.

(a) Mixture of polyethers

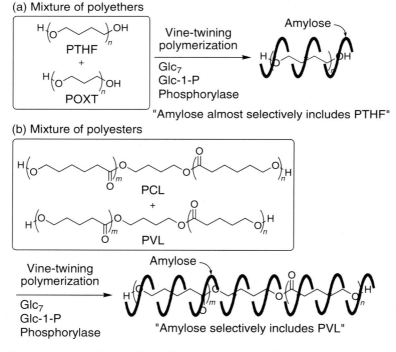

(b) Mixture of polyesters

Figure 8.1 Amylose selectively includes one of the two resemblant polyethers (a) and one of the two resemblant polyesters (b) in vine-twining polymerization.

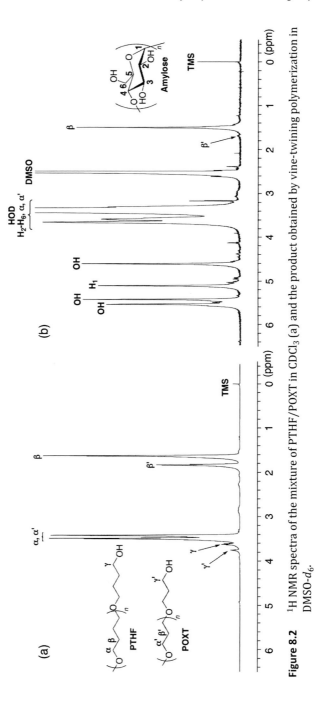

Figure 8.2 ¹H NMR spectra of the mixture of PTHF/POXT in CDCl₃ (a) and the product obtained by vine-twining polymerization in DMSO-d_6.

The concentrations of Glc-1-P and Glc_7 in feed strongly affected the selectivity on the inclusion of amylose in this polymerization manner. When the vine-twining polymerization was carried out in higher concentrations of Glc-1-P and Glc_7 than those described earlier, for example, 15 times, the unit ratio of POXT/PTHF in the products was increased (0.21:1.00) upon increasing the yields of the products (ca. 20 times). Because the concentration of PTHF decreased with the progress of the polymerization due to the predominant inclusion, amylose probably started to include POXT at a later stage of the polymerization.

An attempt of the selective inclusion by amylose in the vine-twining polymerization was also made in the system using the resemblant polyesters (Fig. 8.1b) [2]. The selective inclusion of amylose toward two resemblant polyesters was performed by the vine-twining polymerization in the presence of a mixture of PVL (M_n = 830) and PCL (M_n = 930) under the conditions same as those toward polyethers described earlier. The ^{1}H NMR spectrum of the employed mixture of the guest polyesters (CDCl$_3$) showed that the unit ratio of PVL/PCL in feed was assessed to be 1.00:0.92 (Fig. 8.3a). However, in the ^{1}H NMR spectrum of the product obtained by the vine-twining polymerization (DMSO-d_6), the signals due to PVL and amylose were observed, whereas no signals due to PCL appear (Fig. 8.3b), indicating that amylose has selectively included PVL.

8.1.2 Amylose Selectively Includes a Specific Range of Molecular Weights in Polymers

On the basis of the aforementioned findings, the selective inclusion to a specific range of molecular weights (MWs) in synthetic polymers was investigated by amylose in the vine-twining polymerization because synthetic polymers generally have molecular weight distribution (MWD), meaning that they are reasonably considered as mixtures of analogous molecules with different numbers of the repeating units. Additionally, the number of repeating unit (MW) contributes to show different properties of the polymer with the same structure of repeating unit. For example, PTHF with considerably low MW is soluble in water although PTHF is known as hydrophobic polymer, indicating that the hydrophobicity of PTHF is probably affected by

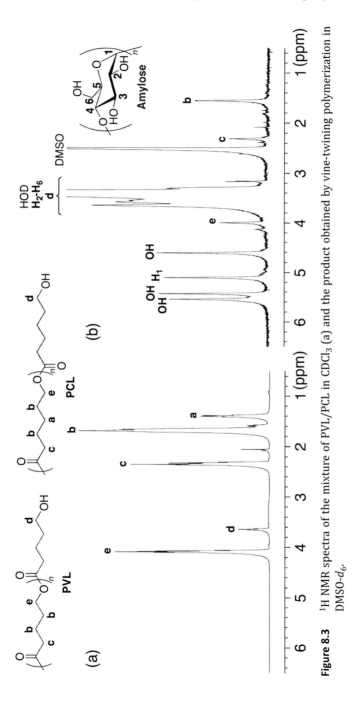

Figure 8.3 ¹H NMR spectra of the mixture of PVL/PCL in CDCl₃ (a) and the product obtained by vine-twining polymerization in DMSO-d_6.

its MW. Therefore, the vine-twining polymerization in the presence of some PTHFs with different average MWs was investigated [4].

The vine-twining polymerization was performed by the phosphorylase-catalyzed enzymatic polymerization of Glc-1-P from Glc_7 in the presence of three PTHFs with different values of M_n and M_w/M_n (PTHF-1K: M_n and M_w/M_n equal to 1350 and 2.86, respectively; PTHF-3K: M_n and M_w/M_n equal to 3040 and 3.13, respectively; and PTHF-6K: M_n and M_w/M_n equal to 6330 and 2.45, respectively) as the guest polymers in sodium acetate buffer at 40–45°C for 6 h (Fig. 8.4a).

To evaluate M_ns and (M_w/M_n)s of PTHFs included in the cavity of amylose, PTHFs were extracted from the inclusion complexes according to the following operation (Fig. 8.4b). After the solutions of the inclusion complexes in DMSO were stirred at 40°C for 13 h, they were added to an excess amount of acetone. Then, the acetone soluble fractions were collected and characterized by ^{1}H NMR measurements to be PTHFs.

The M_ns and (M_w/M_n)s of the extracted PTHFs were estimated by ^{1}H NMR and GPC measurements, respectively. When PTHF-3K with M_w/M_n equal to 3.13 was employed as the guest polymer for the vine-twining polymerization, M_w/M_n of PTHF included in the cavity of amylose became narrow (M_w/M_n = 1.46) although its M_n (=3590) was almost same as that of the employed one (M_n = 3040). These results indicate that amylose selectively included a specific range of MWs in PTHF-3K in the vine-twining polymerization. To investigate the effect of average MWs of the guest PTHFs on the inclusion behavior of amylose, the vine-twining polymerization using PTHF-1K and PTHF-6K as the guest polymers was performed. Consequently, the M_ns and (M_w/M_n)s of PTHFs included in the cavity of amylose were almost same as those using PTHF-3K as mentioned earlier (in the case of using PTHF-1K: M_n and M_w/M_n were equal to 3120 and 1.41, respectively, and using PTHF-6K: M_n and M_w/M_n were equal to 3700 and 1.74, respectively). Thus, it can be concluded that, in this polymerization system, amylose selectively includes a specific range of MWs in PTHFs. These results are probably because of the difference in the inclusion ability of amylose toward PTHFs with various MWs in the vine-twining polymerization.

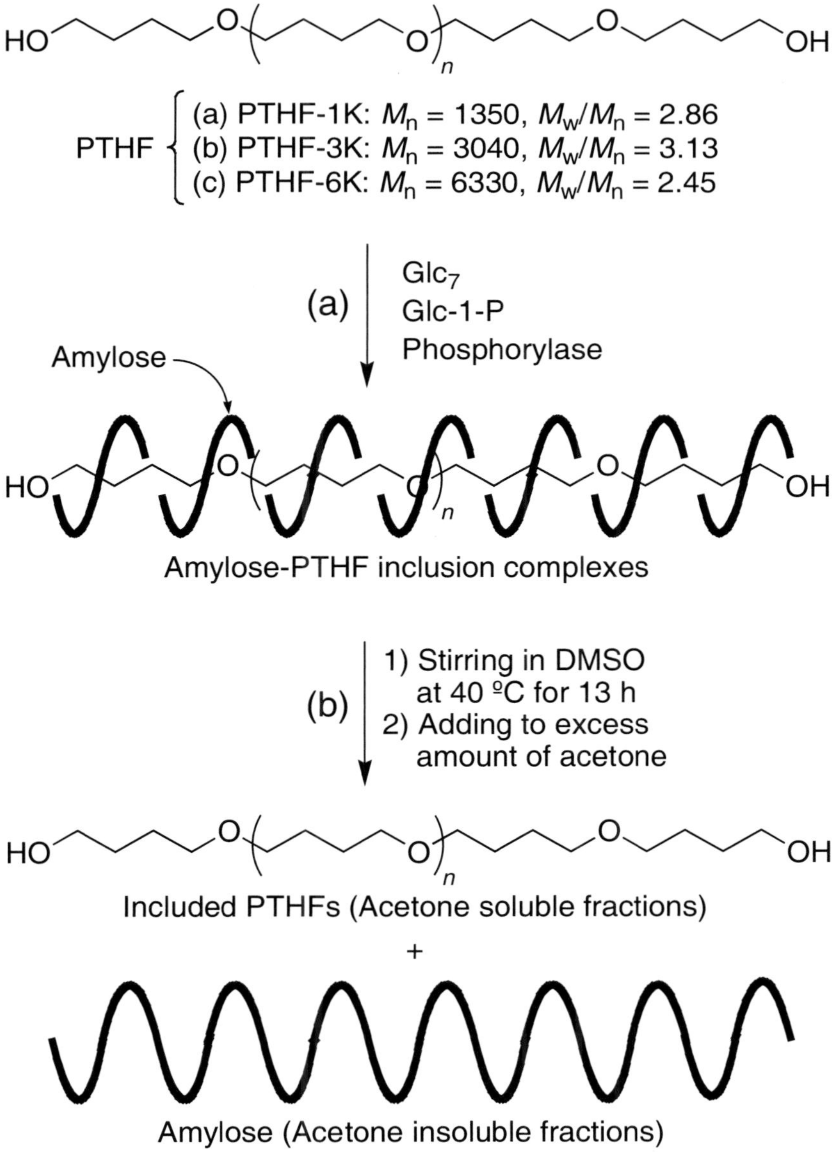

PTHF
{
(a) PTHF-1K: $M_n = 1350$, $M_w/M_n = 2.86$
(b) PTHF-3K: $M_n = 3040$, $M_w/M_n = 3.13$
(c) PTHF-6K: $M_n = 6330$, $M_w/M_n = 2.45$
}

(a) | Glc_7
Glc-1-P
Phosphorylase

Amylose

Amylose-PTHF inclusion complexes

(b) | 1) Stirring in DMSO
at 40 °C for 13 h
2) Adding to excess
amount of acetone

Included PTHFs (Acetone soluble fractions)

+

Amylose (Acetone insoluble fractions)

Figure 8.4 Preparation of amylose–PTHF inclusion complexes by vine-twining polymerization (a) and extraction of PTHFs from the inclusion complexes (b).

8.1.3 Amylose Recognizes Chirality in Poly(lactide)s

Importance of chirality has often appeared in nature because in most cases only one of the enantiomers in the chiral biomolecule exhibits *in vivo* functions in biological systems. For example, in the case of carbohydrates, their D-forms primarily exist in nature and show each specific biological function. Besides such chiral biomolecules, synthetic optically active polymers have also attracted much attention because of various applications such as asymmetric syntheses, chiral adsorbents for separation of racemates in HPLC, and liquid crystals [5]. On the basis of the importance of a sole enantiomer in the aforementioned chiral and optical active functions, a number of chiral recognitions and separations have been performed in the studies on various host–guest systems.

Because amylose is a polysaccharide with left-handed helical (chiral) conformation, it can be considered to be a good candidate for the host molecule that shows ability of chiral recognition toward the optically active polymers such as poly(lactide)s (PLAs) by means of the selective formation of the inclusion complex. Therefore, the recognizable inclusion of amylose toward the chirality in PLAs in the vine-twining polymerization was investigated [6].

First, the vine-twining polymerization was performed by phosphorylase-catalyzed enzymatic polymerization of Glc-1-P from Glc$_7$ in the presence of PLLA (Fig. 8.5a). The precipitated product was characterized by means of the XRD and ^{1}H NMR measurements.

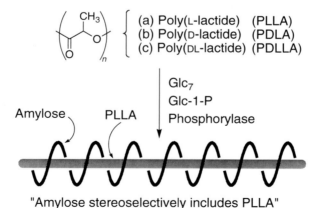

"Amylose stereoselectively includes PLLA"

Figure 8.5 Vine-twining polymerization using phosphorylase in the presence of PLAs.

The XRD pattern of the product obtained from PLLA showed two diffraction peaks at 2θ equal to 11–12° and 18–19° (Fig. 8.6d), which was completely different from that of amylose (Fig. 8.6a) and PLLA (Fig. 8.6b), indicating that the crystalline structure of PLLA was disappeared and the diameter of amylose helix was changed owing to the inclusion of PLLA. Interestingly, the diffraction peaks of the product appeared at lower angles compared with those of the inclusion complexes composed of amylose and the slender guest polymers such as PTHF (2θ = 12–13° and 19–20°) (Fig. 8.6c), as described in Section 7.2 of Chapter 7. The previous studies have reported that one helical turn of amylose is composed of six repeating glucose units when the linear guest molecules of small cross-sectional area are included. However, it has been known that amylose can also include bulky branched alcohols such as isopropyl alcohol, isobutyl alcohol, and *tert*-butyl alcohol to form the corresponding inclusion complexes with the longer helix. Indeed, the XRD patterns of these inclusion complexes, which showed the diffraction peaks at lower angles, i.e., 2θ equal to 11–12° and 18–19°, than those observed

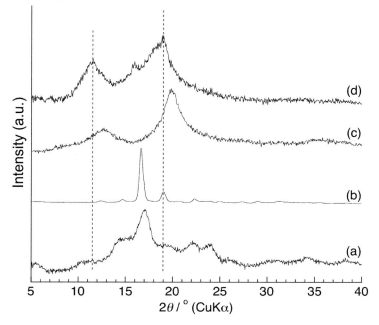

Figure 8.6   XRD patterns of amylose (a), PLLA (b), amylose–PTHF inclusion complex (c), and the product obtained by vine-twining polymerization in the presence of PLLA (d).

in the XRD patterns of the complexes including fatty acids and PTHF, supported the longer diameter of the inclusion complexes. These patterns were similar to those of the product obtained by the vine-twining polymerization using the guest PLLA as described earlier (Fig. 8.6d), indicating the longer diameter of the amylose–PLLA inclusion complex compared with that of the amylose–PTHF inclusion complex, owing to a bulky structure of PLLA due to the branched methyl groups.

The ^{1}H NMR spectrum in DMSO-d_6 of the product obtained from PLLA showed the signals owing to not only amylose but also PLLA, in spite of washing with chloroform as the good solvent for PLLA, indicating that the PLLA was included in the cavity of amylose.

To investigate the effect of the chirality in PLAs on the inclusion of amylose, the vine-twining polymerization was performed using PDLAs (Fig. 8.5b) and PDLLA (Fig. 8.5c) as guests. Consequently, the XRD patterns of the products showed only the diffraction peaks due to amylose (Fig. 8.7) and the ^{1}H NMR spectra did not show the signals due to PLAs, indicating no formation of the corresponding inclusion complexes. These results indicate that amylose perfectly recognized the chirality in PLAs on the formation of inclusion complexes in vine-twining polymerization. The modeling calculations supported the amylose's chiral recognition in favor of PLLA and proposed the atomistic details of the inclusion complex, which involved the preferred orientation of the constituent molecular chains with respect to their fiber axis.

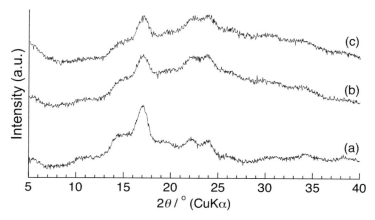

Figure 8.7 XRD patterns of amylose (a) and the products obtained by vine-twining polymerization in the presence of PDLA (b) and PDLLA (c).

8.2 Preparation of Inclusion Complexes Composed of Amylose and Strongly Hydrophobic Polyesters in Parallel Enzymatic Polymerization System

In the vine-twining polymerization as described in Chapter 7, the hydrophobicity of the guest polymers is a very important factor because the driving force for the formation of the inclusion complexes is probably hydrophobic interaction. However, in addition to no formation of the inclusion complex from hydrophilic polymer, e.g., PEG, the preparation of the inclusion complexes had not been achieved from the polymers with strong hydrophobicity, e.g., poly(oxepane), attributed to their aggregation in the aqueous buffer of the solvent for the enzymatic polymerization.

To obtain the inclusion complex from a strongly hydrophobic guest polymer, a parallel enzymatic polymerization system was investigated, i.e., two enzymatic polymerizations, which were the phosphorylase-catalyzed polymerization of Glc-1-P from Glc$_7$, giving rise to amylose, and the lipase-catalyzed polycondensation of dicarboxylic acids and diols, leading to the aliphatic polyesters [7,8], were simultaneously performed (Fig. 8.8) [9]. As the monomers for the guest polyesters, the dicarboxylic acid and the diol having methylene units of 8, hereafter denoted as Diacid-8 and Diol-8, were firstly employed. The isolated product was characterized by means of the ^{1}H NMR and XRD measurements, which supported the structures of amylose–polyester inclusion complex.

To demonstrate that the inclusion complex composed of amylose and the strongly hydrophobic polyester could be prepared by only the present parallel enzymatic polymerization system, following two experiments were performed. First, amylose-forming polymerization was performed in the presence of the polyester having methylene units of 8. In ^{1}H NMR spectrum of the product, the signals due to only amylose were observed, indicating that this polymerization method did not afford corresponding inclusion complex. However, polyester-forming polycondensation was carried out in the presence of amylose. Consequently, although the monomers for the polyester were included in the cavity of amylose, the polyester was not included in it, confirmed by means of ^{1}H NMR measurement. These results indicated that the inclusion complex composed of amylose and the strongly hydrophobic polyester was prepared by only the present parallel enzymatic polymerization system.

$$HOOC-(CH_2)_n-COOH \quad + \quad HO-(CH_2)_n-OH$$

$$\left\{ \begin{array}{l} n = 8; \quad \text{Diacid-8} \\ n = 10; \ \text{Diacid-10} \\ n = 12; \ \text{Diacid-12} \end{array} \right. \qquad \left\{ \begin{array}{l} n = 8; \quad \text{Diol-8} \\ n = 10; \ \text{Diol-10} \\ n = 12; \ \text{Diol-12} \end{array} \right.$$

+

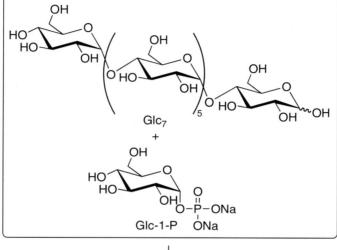

Glc$_7$

+

Glc-1-P

Amylose

Phosphorylase
Lipase

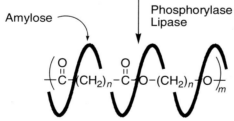

**Inclusion complexes composed of
amylose and strongly hydrophobic polyesters**

Figure 8.8 Preparation of inclusion complexes composed of amylose and strongly hydrophobic polyesters in parallel enzymatic polymerization system.

To investigate the effect of the methylene chain length of the dicarboxylic acids and the diols on the formation of inclusion complexes, the dicarboxylic acids and the diols having methylene units of 10 and 12, hereafter denoted as Diacid-10, Diacid-12, Diol-10, and Diol-12, were employed for this polymerization system. The characterizations of the obtained products were performed by the same manners as those for the product from Diacid-8 and Diol-8 as described earlier. Consequently, it was indicated that the polyesters having methylene units of 10 and 12 were hardly included in the cavity of amylose. Furthermore, the ^{1}H NMR results of the products suggested that relatively larger amounts of Diacid-10 and Diacid-12 were included in the cavity of amylose compared with the case of the inclusion complex obtained using Diacid-8 and Diol-8. Because the hydrophobicities of Diacid-10 and Diacid-12 are stronger than those of Diacid-8, they would be readily included in the cavity of amylose. Actually, when amylose-forming polymerization were investigated in the presence of Diacid-8, Diacid-10, or Diacid-12, individually, the dicarboxylic acids having larger numbers of methylene units were easily included in the cavity of amylose. These results indicated that Diacid-10 and Diacid-12 were predominantly included in the cavity of amylose in the parallel enzymatic polymerization system to disturb the inclusion of the polyesters. In addition, the polyesters obtained using Diacid-10, Diacid-12, Diol-10, and Diol-12 would be aggregated in the aqueous buffer more than those obtained using Diacid-8 and Diol-8 due to stronger hydrophobicity, and accordingly separated from the cavity of amylose.

8.3 Preparation of Hydrogels through the Formation of Inclusion Complex of Amylose

Polymeric hydrogels are three-dimensional polymer networks including a large amount of water, which have been used in a variety of applications because of their high water contents and softness [10]. They are conventionally classified as either chemical or physical gels by the type of cross-linking points. The type of cross-linking structure often determines the properties of the hydrogels.

Because amylose is a biopolymer, it can be enzymatically produced by phosphorylase [11] and hydrolyzed by amylase [12], respectively. Therefore, the hydrogels with cross-linking structure based on amylose have a possibility for the behavior of enzymatic disruption and reproduction of the hydrogels by two enzyme-catalyzed reactions, i.e., the amylase-catalyzed hydrolysis of amylose and the formation of amylose by the phosphorylase-catalyzed polymerization.

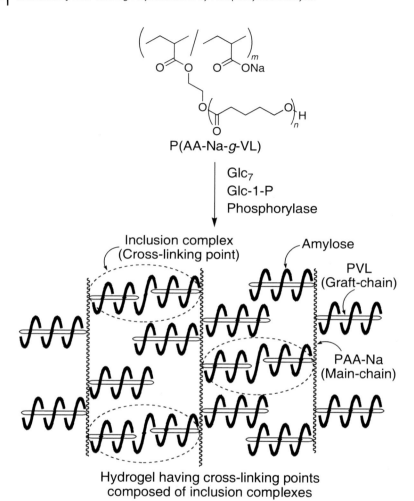

P(AA-Na-*g*-VL)

Glc$_7$
Glc-1-P
Phosphorylase

Inclusion complex
(Cross-linking point)

Amylose

PVL
(Graft-chain)

PAA-Na
(Main-chain)

Hydrogel having cross-linking points
composed of inclusion complexes

Figure 8.9   Preparation of hydrogel by vine-twining polymerization in the presence of poly(acrylic acid sodium salt-*graft*-δ-valerolactone) (P(AA-Na-*g*-VL)).

Therefore, the preparation of hydrogels through the formation of an inclusion complex of amylose in the vine-twining polymerization was investigated [13]. This was achieved by the phosphorylase-catalyzed polymerization of Glc-1-P from Glc$_7$ in the presence of a water-soluble copolymer having the hydrophobic PVL graft chains; poly(acrylic acid sodium salt-*graft*-δ-valerolactone) (P(AA-Na-*g*-VL)) (Fig. 8.9). The enzymatic reaction mixture turned into a gel during

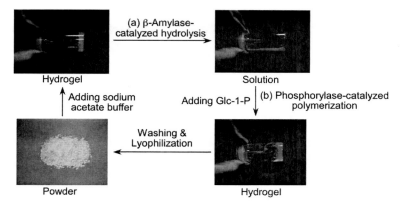

Figure 8.10 Cycle of enzymatic disruption (a) and reproduction of the hydrogel by two enzyme-catalyzed reactions.

the polymerization process. During the enzymatic polymerization, the produced amylose included the PVL graft chains in the intermolecular guest copolymers. Therefore, the formed inclusion complexes acted as the cross-linking points for the formation of the hydrogel. Furthermore, the enzymatic disruption (Fig. 8.10a) and reproduction of the hydrogels (Fig. 8.10b) were achieved by the combination of the β-amylase-catalyzed hydrolysis of the amylose component and the formation of amylose by the phosphorylase-catalyzed polymerization. Therefore, it should be noted that the present hydrogel exhibits the enzymatically recyclable behavior by means of the two enzyme-catalyzed reactions.

References

1. Kaneko, Y., Beppu, K., and Kadokawa, J. (2007). Amylose selectively includes one from a mixture of two resemblant polyethers in vine-twining polymerization, *Biomacromolecules*, **8**, pp. 2983–2985.

2. Kaneko, Y., Beppu, K., Kyutoku, T., and Kadokawa, J. (2009). Selectivity and priority on inclusion of amylose toward guest polyethers and polyesters in vine-twining polymerization, *Polym. J.*, **41**, pp. 279–286.

3. Kadokawa, J., Kaneko, Y., Nagase, S., Takahashi, T., and Tagaya, H. (2002). Vine-twining polymerization: Amylose twines around polyethers to form amylose-polyether inclusion complexes, *Chem. Eur. J.*, **8**, pp. 3321–3326.

4. Kaneko, Y., Beppu, K., and Kadokawa, J. (2009). Amylose selectively includes a specific range of molecular weights in poly(tetrahydrofuran)s in vine-twining polymerization, *Polym. J.*, **41**, pp. 792–796.

5. Yashima, E., Maeda, K., Iida, H., Furusho, Y., and Nagai, K. (2009). Helical polymers: Synthesis, structures, and functions, *Chem. Rev.*, **109**, pp. 6102–6211.

6. Kaneko, Y., Ueno, K., Yui, T., Nakahara, K., and Kadokawa, J. (2011). Amylose's recognition of chirality in polylactides on formation of inclusion complexes in vine-twining polymerization, *Macromol. Biosci.*, **111**, 4308–4345.

7. Kobayashi, S., Uyama, H., Suda, S., and Namekawa, S. (1997). Dehydration polymerization in aqueous medium catalyzed by lipase, *Chem. Lett.*, p. 105.

8. Suda, S., Uyama, H., and Kobayashi, S. (1999). Dehydration polycondensation in water for synthesis of polyesters by lipase catalyst, *Proc. Jpn. Acad. Ser. B: Phys. Biol. Sci.*, **75**, pp. 201–206.

9. Kaneko, Y., Saito, Y., Nakaya, A., Kadokawa, J., and Tagaya, H. (2008). Preparation of inclusion complexes composed of amylose and strongly hydrophobic polyesters in parallel enzymatic polymerization system, *Macromolecules*, **41**, pp. 5665–5670.

10. Lee, K. Y., and Mooney, D. J. (2001). Hydrogels for tissue engineering, *Chem. Rev.*, **101**, pp. 1869–1879.

11. Ziegast, G., and Pfannemüller, B. (1987). Phosphorolytic syntheses with di-, oligo- and multi-functional primers, *Carbohydr. Res.*, **160**, pp. 185–204.

12. Bijttebier, A., Goesaert, H., and Delcour, J. A. (2008). Amylase action pattern on starch polymers, *Biologia*, **63**, pp. 989–999.

13. Kaneko, Y., Fujisaki, K., Kyutoku, T., Furukawa, H., and Kadokawa, J. (2010). Preparation of enzymatically recyclable hydrogels through the formation of inclusion complexes of amylose in a vine-twining polymerization, *Chem. Asian J.*, **5**, pp. 1627–1633.

Chapter 9

Carbohydrate Engineering by Phosphorylase Catalysis

9.1 Facile Synthesis of Glc-1-P from Starch by *Thermus Caldophilus* GK24 Phosphorylase

As described in the previous chapters, phosphorylase is useful for the practical production of amylose, but the problem is that Glc-1-P is expensive. *Thermus caldophilus* GK24 phosphorylase was used to synthesize Glc-1-P from an inexpensive starch [1]. The optimal pH and temperature were 7.0 and 70°C in the phosphorylase reaction with starch producing Glc-1-P. Soluble starch (amylopectin, amylose) turned out to be a better substrate giving a higher yield of Glc-1-P than α-(1→6)-branched α-(1→4)-glucans (glycogen, potato starch, etc.). As a result, Glc-1-P was obtained in a good yield (47%) from the reaction containing 5% soluble starch in 0.7 M potassium phosphate at pH 7.0. Therefore, it can be considered that *T. caldophilus* phosphorylase is readily utilized in large-scale synthesis of Glc-1-P.

9.2 Amylose Production by Combined Use of Phosphorylase with Other Phosphorylases

One possible solution to the expensive problem of Glc-1-P is to combine another enzyme that produces Glc-1-P. Sucrose

Engineering of Polysaccharide Materials: By Phosphorylase-Catalyzed Enzymatic Chain-Elongation
Jun-ichi Kadokawa and Yoshiro Kaneko
Copyright © 2013 Pan Stanford Publishing Pte. Ltd.
ISBN 978-981-4364-45-4 (Hardcover), ISBN 978-981-4364-46-1 (eBook)
www.panstanford.com

phosphorylase catalyzes phosphorolysis of sucrose in the presence of inorganic phosphate (Pi) to produce Glc-1-P and fructose [2,3]. The Glc-1-P thus produced can be used for the phosphorylase-catalyzed synthesis of amylose. When these two enzymatic reactions were individually conducted, the first reaction should be carried out in high concentration of Pi, whereas the Pi should be removed as soon as possible from the media of the second reaction. The combined use of sucrose phosphorylase and phosphorylase in the production of amylose from sucrose was reported by Waldmann et al. (Fig. 9.1) [4]. In this system, interestingly, Pi produced in the second phosphorylase-catalyzed reaction is recycled for the first sucrose phosphorylase-catalyzed reaction. Therefore, the cooperative action by the two phosphorylases proceeds continuously with a constant Pi concentration without any inhibition caused by an accumulation of Pi.

The thermostable sucrose phosphorylase was created by introducing a random and site-directed mutagenesis on the sucrose phosphorylase gene from *Streptococcus mutans* to increase and used together with the triple-mutant phosphorylase (F39L/N135S/T706I) originally from potato for the production of amylose from sucrose [5]. These thermostable variants of sucrose phosphorylase and phosphorylase were employed to optimize the conditions for the production of amylose from sucrose [6,7]. The yields of amylose produced using the two enzymatic catalysis methods from sucrose

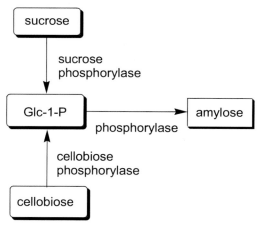

Figure 9.1   Production of amylose by combined use of sucrose or cellobiose phosphorylase and phosphorylase.

were higher than those from Glc-1-P. The molecular weight of amylose was strictly controlled by the sucrose/primer molar ratio. Furthermore, the M_w/M_n of the amylose of all sizes was close to 1, indicating that all the synthesized amylose had a narrow molecular weight distribution, which is same as that of amylose produced using Glc-1-P. The amyloses with molecular weights less than 71×10^3 were produced as insoluble particles, while those with molecular weights more than 305×10^3 were produced in the solution. These results suggested that the properties of amylose differ according to the molecular weights.

For the purpose of providing Glc-1-P, use of cellobiose phosphorylase combined with phosphorylase was also examined (Fig. 9.1). Cellobiose phosphorylase catalyzes a phosphorolytic reaction of cellobiose in the presence of Pi to produce Glc-1-P and glucose [8]. When partially purified cellobiose phosphorylase was incubated with cellobiose and phosphorylase in the presence of Pi, various sizes of amylose (from 4.2×10^4 to 7.3×10^5) were produced [6,7]. However, the yield (38.6%) was not as high as that in the aforementioned method using sucrose phosphorylase. In order to improve the yield of amylose, mutarotase and glucose oxidase were added to the initial reaction mixture [9]. These enzymes were expected to remove the glucose derived by the cellobiose-catalyzed reaction, and thus, shift the equilibrium state to phosphorolysis. The yield of amylose increased to 64.8% by the action of these enzymes. Cellulose is the most abundant biomass resource on the earth, and its effective use is an important research project, leading to the sustainable society in the future. On the basis of this viewpoint, the conversion of cellobiose into amylose is of great interest.

9.3 Synthesis of Branched Glucan by Combined Use of Phosphorylase with Branching Enzyme

Branching enzyme (BE, EC 2.4.1.18) catalyzes transfer of the glucan chain from one α-(1→4)-glucan molecule to a glucan acceptor to form a new α-(1→6)-linkage. The enzyme activity is widely distributed in bacteria, yeasts, plants, and animals, which is responsible for the formation of branching structure in amylopectin and glycogen. The BE genes from several thermophilic microorganisms, such as *B. stearothermphilus* [10] and *Aquifex aeolicus* [11], have been isolated. The BE genes were expressed in various host strains, and the enzymes were well characterized.

Branched glucan can be produced by the combined action of phosphorylase and BE on Glc-1-P in the presence of an adequate primer (Fig. 9.2) [12,13]. The molecular weight and branching pattern of the product are expected to be controlled by the Glc-1-P/primer ratio as in the case of amylose synthesis by the phosphorylase-catalyzed polymerization, and by the relative BE/phosphorylase activity ratio, respectively. Thus, various branched glucans were produced by using different BE/phosphorylase activity ratios. The branched glucans produced at high BE/phosphorylase activity ratios had more frequently branching points than those produced at low BE/phosphorylase ratios.

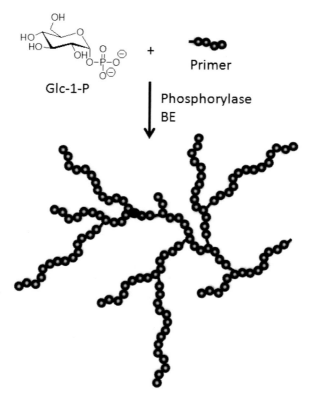

Figure 9.2   Synthesis of branched glucan by combined use of phosphorylase and BE.

Deinococcus geothermalis glycogen branching enzyme is known to catalyze the redistribution of short α-glucans via inter- and intramolecular chain transfer from α-(1→4) positions to α-(1→6) positions. The combined use of phosphorylase and the glycogen branching enzyme gave highly branched amylose from Glc-1-P [14].

References

1. Bae, J., Lee, D., Kim, D., Cho, S. J., Park, J. E., Koh, S., Kim, J., Park, B. H., Choi, Y., Shin, H. J., Hong, S. I., and Lee, D. S. (2005). Facile synthesis of glucose-1-phosphate from starch by *Thermus caldophilus* GK24 α-glucan phosphorylase, *Process Biochem.*, **40**, pp. 3707–3713.

2. Doudoroff, M. (1941). Studies on the phosphorolysis of sucrose, *J. Biol. Chem.*, **151**, pp. 351–361.

3. Taylor, F., Chen, L., Gong, C. S., and Tsao, G. T. (1982). Kinetics of immobilized sucrose phosphorylase, *Biotechnol. Bioeng.*, **24**, pp. 317–328.

4. Waldmann, H., Gygax, D., Bednarski, M. D., Shangraw, R., and Whitesides, G. M. (1986). The enzymic utilization of sucrose in the synthesis of amylose and derivatives of amylose, using phosphorylases, *Carbohydr. Res.*, **157**, pp. c4–c7.

5. Fujii, K., Iiboshi, M., Yanase, M., Takaha, T., and Kuriki. T. (2006). Enhancing the thermal stability of sucrose phosphorylase from *Streptococcus mutans* by random mutagenesis, *J. Appl. Glycosci.*, **53**, pp. 91–97.

6. Yanase, M., Takaha, T., and Kuriki, T. (2006). α-Glucan phosphorylase and its use in carbohydrate engineering, *J. Food Agric.*, **86**, pp. 1631–1635.

7. Ohdan, K., Fujii, K., Yanase, M., Takaha, T., and Kuriki, T. (2006). Enzymatic synthesis of amylose, *Biocatal. Biotransform.*, **24**, pp. 77–81.

8. Ayers, W. A. (1959). Phosphorolysis and synthesis of cellobiose by cell extracts from *Ruminococcus flavefaciens, J. Biol. Chem.*, **234**, pp. 2819–2822.

9. Ohdan, K., Fujii, K., Yanase, M., Takaha, T., and Kuriki, T. (2007). Phosphorylase coupling as a tool to convert cellobiose into amylose, *J. Biotechnol.*, **127**, pp. 496–502.

10. Takata, H., Takaha, T., Kuriki, T., Okada, S., Takagi, M., and Imanaka, T. (1994). Properties and active-center of the thermostable branching

enzyme from bacillus-stearothermophilus, *Appl. Environ. Microbiol.,* **60**, pp. 3096–3104.

11. Takata, H., Ohdan, K., Takaha, T., Kuriki, T., and Okada, S. (2003). Properties of branching enzyme from hyperthermophilic bacterium, *Aquifex aeolicus*, and its potential for production of highly-branched cyclic dextrin, *J. Appl. Glycosci.*, **50**, pp. 15–20.

12. Fujii, K., Takata, H., Yanase, M., Terada, Y., Ohdan, K., Takaha, T., Okada, S., and Kuriki, T. (2003). Bioengineering and application of novel glucose polymers, *Biocatal. Biotransform.*, **21**, pp. 167–172.

13. Kajiura, H., Kakutani, R., Akiyama, T., Takata, H., and Kuriki, T. (2008). A novel enzymatic process for glycogen production, *Biocatal. Biotransform.*, **26**, pp. 133–140.

14. van der Vlist, J., Reixach, M. P., van der Maarel, M., Dijkhuizen, L., Schouten, A. J., and Loos, K. (2008). Synthesis of branched polyglucans by the tandem action of potato phosphorylase and *Deinococcus geothermalis* glycogen branching enzyme, *Macromol. Rapid Commun.*, **29**, pp. 1293–1297.

Chapter 10

Preparation of Amylose-Based Nanomaterials by Phosphorylase Catalysis

10.1 Outlines of Nanomaterials Produced by Self-Assembly or Complex Formation of Macromolecules

Spontaneous self-assembly of macromolecules offers a means to construct a variety of nano-ordered structures. Such nanostructured materials with well-defined shape and size have potential fundamental and practical implications in areas such as materials, supramolecular, and biomimetic chemistries. A typical example for macromolecular self-assembly is provided using block copolymers, wherein different linear homopolymers are linked by covalent bonds [1]. The case of diblock copolymers has been particularly well studied. When diblock copolymers are dissolved in a selective solvent, spontaneous self-assembly into aggregates occurs. Different morphologies will form upon variation of the construction, the quality of the solvent, or the relative length of the two blocks.

However, crystalline amylose–lipid complexes have a V-type structure and can be endogenously present in starch granules [2] or formed upon heating of starch suspensions in the presence of either

Engineering of Polysaccharide Materials: By Phosphorylase-Catalyzed Enzymatic Chain-Elongation
Jun-ichi Kadokawa and Yoshiro Kaneko
Copyright © 2013 Pan Stanford Publishing Pte. Ltd.
ISBN 978-981-4364-45-4 (Hardcover), ISBN 978-981-4364-46-1 (eBook)
www.panstanford.com

endogenous or exogenous lipids [3]. The functionality of emulsifiers in starch-containing systems is often related to complex formation with amylose, and thus, explains the importance of the resultant complexes [4–7].

10.2 Phosphorylase-Catalyzed Synthesis and Molecular Assembly of Amylosic Block Copolymers

Amylosic diblock copolymers were synthesized by phosphorylase-catalyzed polymerization using the polymeric primers having a maltooligosaccharide moiety at the chain end. For example, amylose-*block*-polystyrenes were produced by covalent attachment of maltoheptaose derivatives to end-functionalized polystyrene and subsequent enzymatic polymerization [8–10]. As one of the methods to produce such block copolymers, maltoheptaose was attached by reductive amination to amine-terminated polystyrene (Fig. 10.1) [9]. The phosphorylase-catalyzed polymerization could be started even though the primer-modified polystyrenes were insoluble in citrate buffer of the polymerization medium. The kinetics of the enzymatic polymerization showed an interesting dependence on the molecular weight of polystyrene owing to the micellar structure of the primer in water.

Micellar aggregates of the amylose-*block*-polystyrenes with various compositions were investigated in water and THF using fluorescence correlation spectroscopy, dynamic light scattering (DLS), and asymmetric flow field-flow fractionation with multiangle light-scattering detection [10]. The analytical data indicated the presence of unimers, oligomers, and large micellar species in THF. Up to four different species were detectable by DLS with hydrodynamic radii ranging from a few nanometers to >10 μm, indicating that the system was not in a thermodynamic equilibrium state. Collapsed aggregates were monitored on a silicon surface by scanning force microscopy and transmission electron microscopy. In water, crew-cut micelles were obtained from the same block copolymers by a single-solvent approach, elevated temperature and pressure. These crew-cut aggregates were much more uniform than the respective star aggregates in THF.

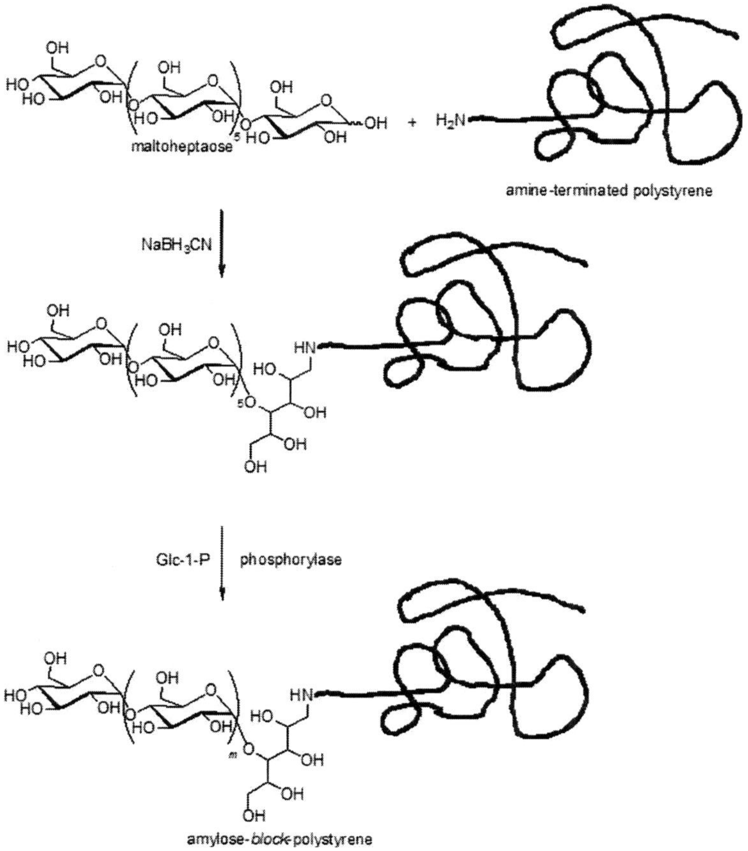

Figure 10.1 Synthesis of amylose-*block*-polystyrene by phosphorylase-catalyzed polymerization.

The synthesis of an amphiphilic methoxy poly(ethylene oxide) (MPEO)-*block*-amylose and its complexation with methyl orange (MO) were investigated [11,12]. First, an MPEO-primer was prepared by the condensation of maltopentanosylamine with MPEO-*p*-nitrophenylcarbonate (Fig. 10.2). Then, the phosphorylase-catalyzed polymerization of Glc-1-P from the primer was carried out to give the MPEO-*block*-amylose. A sole amylose is insoluble in chloroform, but the product was slightly soluble in chloroform. It was confirmed that the complexation of the MPEO-*block*-amylose with MO was significantly enhanced in the amylose domain of the associate in chloroform.

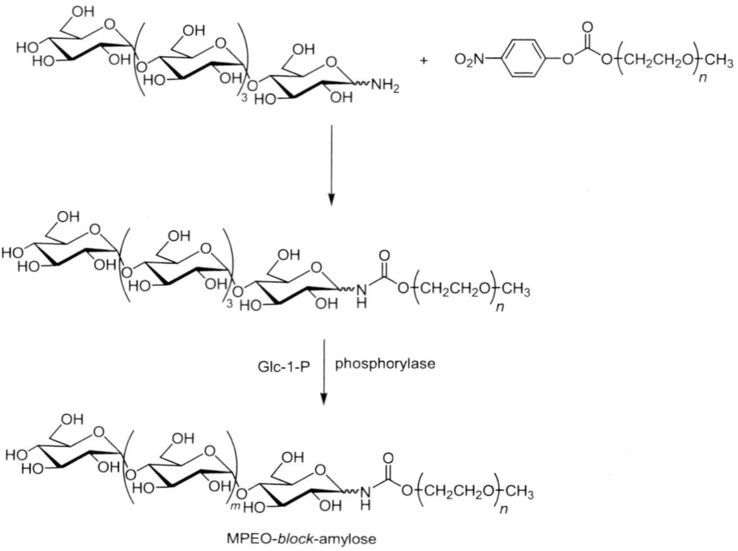

Figure 10.2 Synthesis of MPEO-*block*-amylose by phosphorylase-catalyzed polymerization.

Maltopentaose-*block*-alkyl chain surfactants (C8Glc$_5$, C12Glc$_5$, and C16Glc$_5$) were synthesized, where an alkyl group (C8, C12, and C16) is linked to the reducing end of Glc$_5$ [13,14]. The primers were prepared by the reaction of a Glc$_5$ lactone with octyl-, dodecyl-, or hexadecylamine (Fig. 10.3). The primer surfactants formed micelles in water, which were dissociated upon the phosphorylase-catalyzed polymerization. The enzymatic polymerization of Glc-1-P using the primer surfactants was performed in the presence of phosphorylase b and adenosine 5′-monophosphate sodium salt (AMP) in a Bis–tris buffer at 40°C; this enzyme is activated by AMP. By using the property of the micelle formation of the primer surfactants, the micelle-to-vesicle transition of the mixed lipid/the primer systems was caused by the enzymatic polymerization and could be controlled. Consequently, C12Glc$_5$ micelles were viewed as enzyme-responsive molecular assembly systems. An enzyme-responsive artificial chaperone system using the amphiphilic primer (C12Glc$_5$) as a surfactant and phosphorylase b was designed to enable protein refolding. Effective refolding of carbonic anhydrase B after both heat denaturation (70°C for 10 min) and guanidine hydrochloride (6 M) denaturation was observed by controlled association between the protein molecules and the C12Glc$_5$ primer micelle through the enzymatic polymerization.

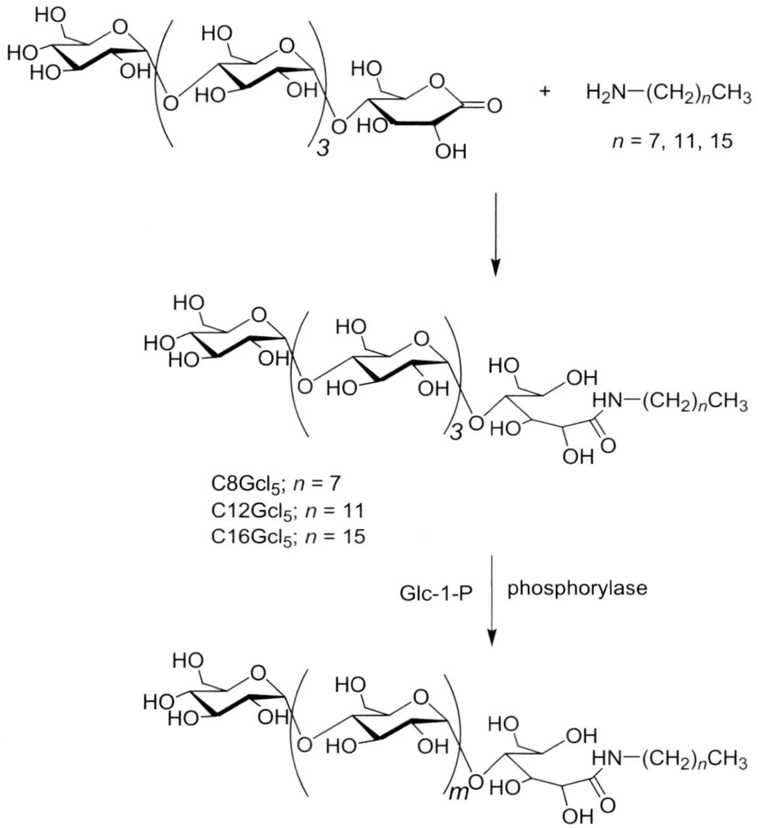

Figure 10.3 Synthesis of maltopentaose-*block*-alkyl chain surfactants and use as primers for phosphorylase-catalyzed polymerization.

10.3 Formation of Amylose–Lipid Complexes through Phosphorylase-Catalyzed Polymerization

During the phosphorylase-catalyzed polymerization of Glc-1-P using maltohexaose in the presence of lipids, amylose–lipid complexes were spontaneously formed and precipitated [15]. They were recovered by centrifugation and lyophilization, and characterized by X-ray diffraction and differential scanning calorimetry. The presence of lipids during the amylose synthesis led to lower amylose DP.

Lipid chain length defined amylose DP, which increased in the order myristic acid (C14), glyceryl monostearate (GMS), stearic acid (C18), and docosanoic acid (C22). The thermal stability of the complexes increased in the same manner, with C22 complexes having the highest dissociation temperature [15,16].

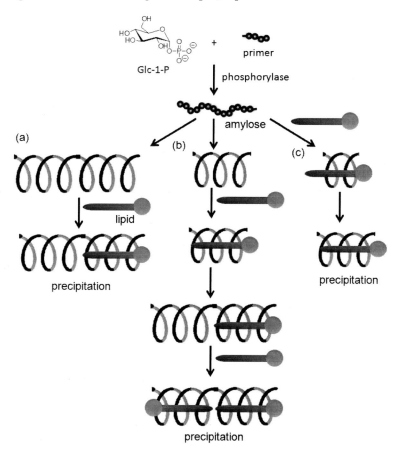

Figure 10.4 Possible mechanisms of the semienzymic synthesis of amylose–lipid complexes. (a) Complexation and precipitation only when amylose chain is long enough; (b) complexation after a small amylose chain is formed, further elongation of the amylose and subsequent complexation, precipitation occurs when a sufficient number of lipids are complexed; (c) "vine-twining": amylose synthesis around lipid, with precipitation when a sufficient number of lipid molecules are complexed.

A further study revealed that the phosphorylase dosage and Glc-1-P/primer ratio influenced the reaction rate of the enzymatic synthesis, presumably by changing the balance between amylose synthesis and amylose–lipid complexation and precipitation, and impacted the molecular weight of the complexes [17]. Tailor-made short-chain amylose–lipid complexes could be produced by choosing the appropriate reaction conditions. In general, several interactions between the growing amylose chains and the lipids can be envisaged. First, enzymatic synthesis and complexation/precipitation occur rather independently, i.e., resembling classical synthesis (Fig. 10.4a). Complexation and precipitation would only take place after a longer amylose chain has been synthesized. It is also possible that amylose is synthesized around the lipid present, resulting in immediate complexation, while precipitation only occurs when a sufficient number of lipids are incorporated in the amylose helix (vine-twining complexation, Fig. 10.4c).

An intermediate between these two as a way was proposed, in which amylose–lipid complexes are synthesized semienzymatically (Fig. 10.4b); elongation of the primer occurs until an amylose chain is obtained that is sufficiently long to complex at least one lipid molecule. This complex then stays in the solution and the enzymatic chain extension of the amylose chain continues, together with the subsequent complexation, until the formed amylose–lipid complex becomes insoluble and precipitates.

References

1. Kim, J. K., Yang, S. Y., Lee, Y., and Kim, Y. (2010). Functional nanomaterials based on block copolymer self-assembly, *Prog. Polym. Sci.*, **35**, pp. 1325–1349.

2. Morrison, W. R. (1988). Lipids in cereal starches: A review, *J. Cereal Sci.*, **8**, pp. 1–15.

3. Morrison, W. R., Law, R. V., and Snape, C. E. (1993). Evidence for inclusion complexes of lipids with V-amylose in maize, rice and oat starches, *J. Cereal Sci.*, **18**, pp. 107–109.

4. Eliasson, A. C., and Ljunger, G. (1988). Interactions between amylopectin and lipid additives during retrogradation in a model system, *J. Sci. Food Agric.*, **44**, pp. 353–361.

5. Gudmundsson, M., and Eliasson, A. C. (1990). Retrogradation of amylopectin and the effects of amylose and added surfactants emulsifiers, *Carbohydr. Polym.*, **13**, pp. 295–315.

6. Gudmundsson, M. (1992). Effects of an added inclusion-amylose complex on the retrogradation of some starches and amylopectin, *Carbohydr. Polym.*, **17**, pp. 299–304.

7. Goesaert, H., Brijs, K., Veraverbeke, W. S., Courtin, C. M., Gebruers, K., and Delcour, J. A. (2005). Wheat flour constituents: How they impact bread quality, and how to impact their functionality, *Trends Food Sci. Technol.*, **16**, pp. 12–30.

8. Loos, K., and Stadler, R. (1997). Synthesis of amylose-*block*-polystyrene rod-coil block copolymers, *Macromolecules*, **30**, pp. 7641–7643.

9. Loos, K., and Müller, A. H. E. New routes to the synthesis of amylose-*block*-polystyrene rod-coil block copolymers, *Biomacromolecules*, **3**, pp. 368–373.

10. Loos, K., Böker, A., Zettl, H., Zhang, M., Krausch, G., and Müller, A. H. E. *Macromolecules*, **38**, pp. 873–879.

11. Akiyoshi, K., Kohara, M., Ito, K., Kitamura, S., and Sunamoto, J. (1999). Enzymatic synthesis and characterization of amphiphilic block copolymers of poly(ethylene oxide) and amylose, *Macromol. Rapid Commun.*, **20**, pp. 112–115.

12. Akiyoshi, K., Maruichi, N., Kohara, M., and Kitamura, S. (2002). Amphiphilic block copolymer with a molecular recognition site: Induction of a novel binding characteristic of amylose by self-assembly of poly(ethylene oxide)-*block*-amylose in chloroform, *Biomacromolecules*, **3**, pp. 280–283.

13. Morimoto, N., Ogino, N., Narita, T., Kitamura, S., and Akiyoshi, K. (2007). Enzyme-responsive molecular assembly system with amylose-primer surfactants, *J. Am. Chem. Soc.*, **129**, pp. 458–459.

14. Morimoto, N., Ogino, N., Narita, T., and Akiyoshi, K. (2009). Enzyme-responsive artificial chaperone system with amphiphilic amylose primer, *J. Biotechnol.*, **140**, pp. 246–249.

15. Gelders, G. G., Goesaert, H., and Delcour, J. A. (2005). Potato phosphorylase catalyzed synthesis of amylose-lipid complexes, *Biomacromolecules*, **6**, pp. 2622–2629.

16. Gelders, G. G., Goesaert, H., and Delcour, J. A. (2006). Amylose-lipid complexes as controlled lipid release agents during starch gelatinization and pasting, *J. Agric. Food Chem.*, **54**, pp. 1493–1499.

17. Putseys, J. A., Derde, L. J., Lamberts, L., Goesaert, H., and Delcour, J. A. (2009). Production of tailor made short chain amylose–lipid complexes using varying reaction conditions, *Carbohydr. Polym.*, **78**, pp. 854–861.

Index

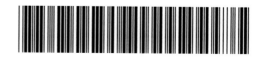